The
Hormone
Survival
Guide
for

PERIMENOPAUSE

Balance Your Hormones Naturally

D1015234

"This is a great book, giving women concrete actions and guidelines for managing their own health."

George Gillson, M.D., Ph.D.
Author of You've Hit Menopause: Now What?

"One of the best choices available on the subject of perimenopause. Easy to follow and understand..."

Jim Paoletti, R.Ph., FIACP
Professional Compounding Centers of America

"Easy to read and very informative."

Jennifer R. Berman, M.D.
Female Sexual Medicine Center at UCLA
Author of For Women Only: A Revolutionary Guide to Reclaiming Your Sex Life

"Never before have I found a health book that is so accessible and easily understandable. Since I put Dr. Jackson's methods into effect, the results have been truly amazing. I've got more energy, have lost weight, and look and feel better than I have in years."

Beth R.
Patient, age 41

"In all my years of doing talk radio and covering the sensitive topic of women's emotions and the men who don't understand them, I have not come across a book as practical and helpful as this one."

Perry Atkinson
General Manager
KDOV Radio

The
Hormone
Survival
Guide
for
PERIMENOPAUSE

Balance Your Hormones Naturally

Nisha Jackson, Ph.D.

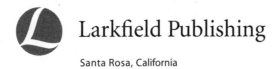

Larkfield Publishing

Santa Rosa, California

Publisher: Gary Palmatier
Developmental Editor: Mary Korbulic
Copy Editor: Elizabeth von Radics
Proofreader: Susan Gall
Indexer: Edwin Durbin
Cover Designer: Ideas to Images
Cover Photographer: Christopher Briscoe
Compositor and Illustrator: Ideas to Images

Larkfield Publishing
5256 Aero Drive, Unit 3
Santa Rosa, CA 95403
(707) 542-9057
(707) 542-9056 fax
www.larkfieldpublishing.com

All trademarks and registered trademarks mentioned herein are the property of their respective holders.

Printed in Canada

Publisher's Cataloging-in-Publication Data
Jackson, Nisha.
    The hormone survival guide for perimenopause :
balance your hormones naturally / Nisha Jackson.
    p. cm.
    Includes bibliographical references and index.
    LCCN 2003111292
    ISBN 0-9742067-0-9
    1. Perimenopause—Hormone therapy.   2. Perimenopause
—Alternative treatment—Popular works.   I. Title.

    RG188.J33 2004   618. 1'7506
                                             QB103-200662

Contents

Foreword by Neal Rouzier, M.D.   *xiii*

Preface   *xv*

Important Caution to the Reader   *xviii*

Introduction   1

To Test or Not to Test?   2

Why I Wrote This Book   4

How This Book Can Help   5

CHAPTER 1

Why Hormonal Chaos?   7

Current Medical Thinking About Hormones   8

The Hormone Roller Coaster   8

Hormones and Aging: Decline and Confusion   10

Hormone Levels Decline with Age   10

What Is Perimenopause and
Why Do I Have to Go Through It?   12

CHAPTER 2

Know Your Hormones
in and out of Balance   15

Perimenopause: The Change Before the Change   16

How Do Hormones Tip out of Balance?   17

The Hormonal Domino Effect   18

Hormonal Highs and Lows   19

Estrogen   19

    What Is Estrogen Dominance?   *21*

Progesterone   23

The Benefits of Progesterone   24

    What Happens When Progesterone Levels Drop?   *24*

Testosterone   25

CHAPTER   3

Have Your Hormones Tested   27

Why Test Your Hormones?   28

    Each Woman Is Unique   *28*

    Bucking the Trend   *29*

Timing Is Everything   31

Testing Options   31

    Serum (Blood) Testing   *31*

Serum-Testing Specifics   32

    Saliva Testing   *34*

    Urine Testing   *34*

Interpreting Lab Results   34

Saliva-Testing Specifics   35

    Estradiol   *36*

    Testosterone   *38*

Working with Your Medical Provider   38

Long-term Hormonal Balance   39

CHAPTER 4

Use Hormones to Treat Hormone Problems 41

Natural Versus Synthetic Hormones 42

Individualizing Hormone Treatment 44

How to Use Progesterone 45

Progesterone Versus Synthetic Progesterone (Progestin) 45

Forms of Natural Progesterone 46

Administering Progesterone 47

Dosages of Natural Progesterone 47

How Do I Know If I Need Progesterone? 48

What to Expect When Using Progesterone 49

Troubleshooting: Progesterone 49

Estrogen Therapy in Perimenopause 50

When Is Estrogen Helpful? 50

Natural Estrogen Choices 52

Dosages of Natural Estrogen 53

Synthetic Estrogen Alternatives 53

Additional Alternatives for Correcting Estrogen Balance 54

How to Use Estrogen While Still Having Periods 54

Liver Flush Cocktail 56

What About Testosterone? 57

Things to Remember When Using Testosterone Replacement 58

Dosages of Testosterone 59

Moving Forward with Hormonal Balance 59

CHAPTER   5

Fix Your Diet: The Most Powerful Way to Create Hormonal Balance   61

Why Women Gain Weight with Age   62

A Six-Step Plan for Weight/Fat Loss   64

Step 1: Eat Protein   64

High-Protein, Low-Fat Snacks   65

Step 2: Eliminate Sugar   65

High-Protein, Healthy Snacks   65

Step 3: Eat Your Fruits and Veggies   66

Many-Veggie Soup   66

Salad Tips   67

Salad Dressing: The Silent Saboteur   67

Step 4: Drink Water   68

Step 5: Incorporate "Good Fat"   68

Yogurt Cream Cheese   68

Step 6: Get Moving!   69

Tips for Success   69

Simple Steps to Support Your Efforts   70

Supplements for Weight/Fat Loss   71

Exercise Your Way to a Lean Body   72

CHAPTER   6

Eliminate the Stress Hormone   75

The Story of Stress   76

The Overworked Adrenal Glands   77

Where Things Go Wrong for the Busy Woman 77

  Solutions for the Stressed-out Busy Woman 80

Signs of Toxic Stress 80

Solutions for Resolving Toxic Stress 80

  Solutions for the Working Woman 81

Supplements for Stress Management 82

  General Solutions for Every Woman 84

Diet for Toxic Stress 85

The Quick-Fix Plan for Stress 86

Exercise for Toxic Stress 86

C H A P T E R 7

Get a Grip on PMS 87

PMS During Perimenopause 88

What Causes PMS? 89

Factors Increasing the Incidence and Severity of PMS 91

Diagnosing PMS 91

  PMS Assessment 91

PMS Treatment Options 93

  Steps You Can Take on Your Own 93

Guidelines for the Hypoglycemia Diet 94

  Supplements 94

  Progesterone Therapy 95

Recommended Options for Progesterone Therapy 96

  Antidepressants 96

CHAPTER 8

Turn on Your Sex Drive   97

Is Losing Libido Inevitable?   98

Did You Know...?   99

What Is a "Healthy" Sex Drive?   99

Foods to Fuel the Fire   100

Hormones to Increase Sex Drive   101

Hormone Therapy   102

Alternatives for Improving Sex Drive   103

Simple Exercises for Improved Body Image   105

Additional Sex-Drive Blasters   106

Simple Ways to Spice Up Your Love Life   107

A Dream Date at Home   108

CHAPTER 9

The Fatigue Factor:
Rejuvenate Your Thyroid   109

The Powerful Thyroid   110

Low Thyroid Is a Common Complaint   110

Undiagnosed, Untreated Low Thyroid Is Bad News   111

Why Is Low Thyroid So Often Undiagnosed?   111

Low Thyroid in Perimenopause   112

Symptoms of Low Thyroid   113

Other Causes of Fatigue   113

Testing for Thyroid Disorders   116

Obtaining an Accurate Diagnosis   117

Treatment Options   118

What About Osteoporosis?   118

Which Treatment Is Most Effective?   120

Natural Supplements for Hypothyroidism   120

The Quick-Fix Plan for Energy   121

CHAPTER   10

Other Hazards of Perimenopause   123

Surviving Hot Flashes and Night Sweats   124

Factors Under Your Control   124

Supplements for Regulating Hot Flashes and Night Sweats   125

What Can I Do About Irregular Periods?   127

Hope for Thinning Hair and Hair Loss   129

Hair 101   129

Diet, Exercise, and Stress Reduction   129

Supplements   130

Prescription Medications   130

Hair-care Products   131

Banishing Breast Tenderness   131

The Cure for Vaginal Dryness and Irritation   133

Hormone Treatments   133

Treating Migraines and Other Headaches   134

Preventive Measures for Headaches   136

Bladder Control 101   137

Getting a Good Night's Sleep   138

Why Is Sleep So Important?   138

Establishing Better Sleep Patterns   139

EPILOGUE

The 12-Week
Hormone-Balancing Plan

141

The 12-Week Hormonal Overhaul   142

The 12-Week Diet Overhaul   143

De-Stressing   144

The Six-Step Plan for Jumpstarting Energy   144

You Can Do It   145

Appendix A: Compounding Pharmacies
and Hormone-Testing Laboratories   147

Appendix B: Vitamin and
Herbal Supplement Resources   149

Appendix C: Products   151

Appendix D: Recommended Reading
for Specific Perimenopausal Problems   152

Appendix E: Bibliography   155

Glossary   164

Index   169

Foreword

by Neal Rouzier, M.D.

As a physician specializing in natural hormones, I am constantly working with people who are looking for answers. They are frustrated with the changes taking place in their bodies and their feelings of being out of control. Women in the premenopause years—thirty-five to fifty—commonly suffer from such symptoms as acne, bloating, depression, exhaustion, insomnia, weight gain, joint pain, facial hair, food cravings, fuzzy thinking, and loss of sex drive. They are discouraged by their current physicians telling them there is nothing wrong, that it's "normal," or to "just learn to live with it." More and more women are no longer willing to settle for feeling bad. They are discovering that symptom control and even symptom alleviation are within their grasp—without resorting to animal-based synthetic hormone treatments that have been shown to have potentially dangerous side effects.

If you are reading this book, you are one of those women who are looking for a better option. You are taking the initiative to research the answer to the question *Do I really have to feel like this?* This book answers that question—and many others—by showing you that the commonly perceived notion of perimenopause is just that: a notion. You really can feel and look fantastic at thirty-five, fifty, and beyond. Being armed with this enlightening information could be essential to your quality of life.

As you read this book, it is important to understand that it's not really your physician's fault that he or she is largely unaware of natural hormone therapy or the control you can have over your perimenopausal symptoms. The average physician is simply taught to treat a sickness or an injury. Menopause—and the hormonal decline that accompanies it—is not considered a disease but a natural course of life. If you asked a perimenopausal woman if she feels "normal" and happy, however, most often the answer would be *NO!*

Dr. Nisha Jackson has done an excellent job of understanding the health-care plight of the perimenopausal woman and how to get out of the healthcare cycle of disease. She gives you guidelines on how you can take control of your symptoms and your life.

The challenge for practitioners with a holistic/functional/integrative approach is to step back and look at the big picture: What are the ways to fine-tune a body entering middle age? The global view of healthy aging or preventive medicine takes us far beyond conventional medicine and becomes a challenge for us all: Don't just treat the symptoms; strengthen the body so it can put up a good fight.

Dr. Jackson explains and teaches you how to do just that—through diet, exercise, stress reduction, and natural hormone supplements. I believe you will benefit tremendously from her expertise and guidance. After you have finished, be sure to tell a friend about this book and how it changed your life!

Preface

Too many self-help books for hormonally unbalanced women do not seem to appreciate that women in crisis do not want sift through hundreds of pages of medical jargon. Women experiencing extreme PMS or premenopausal madness need answers and help as quickly as possible. So let's get started!

I begin the book with an introduction that tells how it came about and how I hope it can help you. Chapters 1 and 2 give you important background information on hormones, perimenopause, and the profound effects of hormonal decline and imbalance. Then we really get down to the business of what you can do about feeling better *now*.

The 7-Step Program to Balance Your Hormones

Chapters 3 through 9 are devoted to the seven steps I have identified that women can take to gain control of their lives:

▶ **Step 1:** Have your hormones tested

▶ **Step 2:** Use hormones to treat hormone problems

▶ **Step 3:** Fix your diet

▶ **Step 4:** Eliminate the stress hormone

▶ **Step 5:** Get a grip on PMS

▶ **Step 6:** Turn on your sex drive

▶ **Step 7:** Rejuvenate your thyroid

In each chapter I explain clearly and concisely why each step is important, the symptoms it addresses, the pitfalls you should avoid, and the beneficial results you can expect.

You can choose to read the chapters in order—each step is important to your success in correcting the potentially devastating effects of hormonal imbalance—or you may want to skip around and read those chapters that discuss the particular challenges you are currently facing.

Chapter 10 describes other common health problems that women face as they enter their middle years—and the solutions that are available.

The book ends with several appendices full of resources and recommended reading, a glossary defining the key words you'll need to know when talking to your healthcare professional, and a comprehensive index.

Acknowledgments

I offer my deepest gratitude for the opportunity to write this book. The process of bringing it to you was in no way solitary, and I owe many thanks to all of the patients and pioneers in the field of hormonal balance who inspired me to write a book that women can use to positively guide them in their journey through the perimenopause years.

Grateful thanks go to my colleagues who reviewed the book and provided valuable input: Perry Atkinson, Dr. Jennifer Berman, Dr. George Gillson, Jim Paoletti, Carol Petersen, Dr. Neal Rouzier, and Larry Thorne.

I am indebted to my publisher, Gary Palmatier, who not only had the vision to see what this book could become and the women whose lives could benefit from it, but also believed in me and my mission to see this through.

I received invaluable help in the preparation of the manuscript from friend and developmental editor Mary Korbulic, whose deep understanding and verbal artistry helped me shape my thoughts into words.

Thank you, thank you to Elizabeth von Radics, my copyeditor, for meticulously running her fine-toothed comb over the manuscript and keeping me grammatically correct and for always smiling and staying positive. Thanks also to proofreader Susan Gall for her careful work and to Barbara Moller for her wonderful recipes. And a thank-you to photographer Christopher Briscoe for his keen eye and cool professionalism at a moment's notice.

I am also indebted to Perry Atkinson at KDOV for providing me with my regular radio show, which allows me to teach multitudes of women that taking care of oneself is so important.

Many thanks to my mother, who taught me to truly care for people, and to my father, who gave me my drive and taught me to never give up! Humble thanks to my wonderful staff, who always believe in me and push me to bring my best forward.

Thanks also to my friends, each of whom offered her unique support during this time of writing, especially Shannon, Dayna, Shari, Sandi, Jeannie, Lisa, Judi, and Peggy, and to my partners, Dan, Beverly, and Julie.

And thank you to Rick, Jordan, and McKenzie—my three most treasured companions, my biggest fans, and my most loyal supporters. I owe them so much for hanging in there with me throughout this project; I am most truly blessed to have them in my life.

Finally, I hope that in reading this book you will recognize the gratitude that I have toward all of the patients who have shared their lives with me to bring this book to you. To God be all of the glory that comes from this book.

Nisha Jackson

Important Caution to the Reader

This book is not intended to take the place of advice, supervision, and care from medical and other healthcare professionals and should not be used as a substitute for obtaining such services from qualified practitioners. Neither the author nor the publisher is giving medical, psychological, or nutritional advice or otherwise rendering medical, psychological, or nutritional services.

As noted above, readers should consult an appropriate medical or other healthcare professional before using or relying on any of the advice, information, comments, or other content of this book. Proper medical advice and supervision are especially important *before* making decisions about exercise, diet, nutrition, supplements, medication, testing, and other health issues.

This book is published, distributed, and sold without warranties or guarantees of any kind, express or implied; and the author and publisher disclaim any responsibility or liability for any loss, damage, or other consequences resulting directly or indirectly from any use of this publication or the information, advice, or other content of this book.

Introduction

Women in ever-increasing numbers are seeking alternatives to traditional healthcare—and for good reason. Imagine a woman between thirty-five and fifty. A spare tire is developing around her middle, and bags have made unwelcome appearances beneath her eyes. Hot flashes come and go throughout the day, and night sweats interrupt her sleep. She is exhausted, can't seem to concentrate, and alternates between depression and flying off the handle. Upset and anxious, she seeks help for the unpleasant physical and emotional changes that are crowding the good times out of her life.

After a physical exam and a few questions, to her dismay her medical provider suggests that what she's going through is perfectly normal: She is simply approaching the time when her periods will cease—*menopause*—and the disagreeable symptoms she is experiencing are part and parcel of getting older. Her doctor may mention that she is probably in *perimenopause,* the years leading up to menopause, during which hormones fluctuate and birth control pills or hormone replacement therapy (HRT) may be prescribed. If the woman is depressed, she may be sent to the pharmacy for a bottle of Prozac or other prescription antidepressant. Or perhaps her provider, judging her to be just another hysterical female, proposes that all she *really* needs is to "get her stress under control and lose some weight," then sends her on her not-so-merry way.

If this sounds familiar, you may be one of the multitudes of women whose perimenopausal symptoms have either been dismissed as a natural consequence of aging and/or treated with conventional therapies. A growing number of women are no longer willing to be dismissed or accept standard treatment. Armed with information from books such as this, they are demanding a level of care that their mothers could not have imagined. It is personalized, one-on-one female care that considers the whole woman in her physical, emotional, and *hormonal* aspects. This care gives a woman her best shot at conquering current health problems and staving off future ills. Perhaps best of all, it helps her avoid unnecessary or unsafe medications that don't provide long-term solutions to hormonal imbalances.

If you have been prescribed drugs containing synthetic hormones, and you use the medications as directed, chances are the results haven't been what you had hoped. Your hot flashes may be gone, your periods may return to regularity, but you may also experience a spectrum of negative side effects, including bloating, irregular bleeding, sore breasts, and weight gain. Like millions of American women, you are using powerful hormone medications prescribed by healthcare practitioners who have no way of knowing your hormone levels! You are getting a one-size-fits-all treatment that does not address the list of maladies that can accompany hormonal imbalances. This long list includes bloating, depression, exhaustion, acne, insomnia, weight gain, facial hair, food cravings, fuzzy thinking, joint pain, and loss of sex drive. Although some perimenopausal women tolerate synthetic hormones such as those found in birth control pills and HRT, others experience mild to severe side effects that can be more annoying or debilitating than the symptoms they are meant to relieve.

Does this mean that women should not take hormones? No. But it does mean that women must educate themselves about the differences between synthetic and natural hormones and make informed choices.

Using any type of drug, including natural hormones, is not the first course of action, however. Many perimenopausal symptoms can be relieved through a combination of lifestyle modifications, stress reduction, and use of supplements. So how do we know if our hormones, particularly estrogen, progesterone, and testosterone, are in balance? We gauge their levels with reliable lab tests so that accurate dosing and treatment decisions can relieve symptoms and create hormonal balance.

To Test or Not to Test?

It sounds like a no-brainer that hormone testing should be routine, but for several reasons testing is the exception rather than the rule. First, it is not "standard of care" or deemed medically necessary. This means that when you have a problem that may be related to your cycle and the hormone fluctuations that go with it, your medical provider is not required to order a test to measure your hormone levels before you are treated. Instead, he or she can prescribe birth control pills or synthetic HRT at any time, with only subjective information or a hunch that these drugs may be right for you.

The reasons why hormone testing—and prescribing natural hormones—is not standard of care has more to do with patent law and the pharmaceutical industry than anything else. There is also the fact that most medical schools have until recently ignored natural hormones as an option in treating women's hormonal imbalances. But let's go back to the drug companies. Natural, plant-based hormones cannot be patented and marketed as exclusive products. Even though safe, plant-based sources for making bioidentical natural progesterone and estrogen are readily available, pharmaceutical companies rarely use them (although the discrediting of synthetic hormones is beginning to propel them in that direction). Instead they use lab-formulated synthetic progestins and estrogens to make their HRT formulas. When sales representatives talk with doctors, they offer flashy brochures and literature about double-blind studies conducted and/or financed, of course, by the drug companies. For some drugs—*ever heard of Celebrex or Viagra?*—manufacturers appeal directly to consumers, who in turn request that their healthcare providers prescribe these drugs.

Nobody is pitching natural hormones to medical offices because, at least for now, there is no fortune to be made. In fact, mainstream healthcare providers who are familiar enough with natural hormones to prescribe them are in the minority. So it is no surprise that mainstream medical practitioners are reluctant to initiate hormone testing to determine dosing for medicines they know little or nothing about.

The same goes for natural supplements and herbal remedies. These alternatives have neither private funding nor representatives hounding medical offices to tout their benefits. If medical providers want to find out about these alternatives, they must do just as you are doing—educate themselves. Given their hectic schedules, time constraints, and demanding practices, it isn't too surprising that most healthcare practitioners haven't done so.

I think it will all come around, however, because patients are going to demand it—if they aren't already. Women are justifiably scared of synthetic HRT, and word is getting out that therapy using natural, bioidentical hormones is a safe and effective alternative for relieving unpleasant symptoms.

Medical practitioners who lack education about hormone testing and treatment with the natural alternatives nevertheless claim that hormone testing is inaccurate because levels change constantly as a woman cycles through the month. Hormone levels *do* fluctuate, and every woman *is* unique, but those facts don't cancel the value and accuracy of carefully conducted hormone testing. It is being done successfully and has been absolutely invaluable in my medical practice and those of informed colleagues across the nation.

Women come to me with a multitude of complaints, and I have found that testing at the appropriate time, interpreting the results, and moving forward with effective therapies are the cornerstones of care. Whether through blood or saliva, testing is an excellent way to pinpoint hormone levels as women enter the perimenopausal years.

Consider a forty-three-year-old patient who has missed some periods and has perimenopausal symptoms, such as hot flashes, headaches, night sweats, insomnia, mood changes, and weight gain. Her medical provider orders the widely used FSH (follicle-stimulating hormone) test, which indicates that she is not in menopause. She is advised to come back next year for another FSH test. Such testing helps determine whether a woman is nearing menopause, but it is notoriously inaccurate and at any rate does not provide information on individual hormone levels. So the poor woman is condemned to her unpleasant symptoms for another year because one questionable test says so.

On the other hand, had the provider ordered a complete hormone panel, it probably would have revealed that the woman's hormone levels were either low or out of balance. Knowing a woman's estrogen, progesterone, testosterone, DHEA (dehydroepiandrosterone), and thyroid levels would not only allow for a customized treatment plan to relieve her symptoms, but also provide a baseline to observe changes as she moves through perimenopause to menopause. Testing allows an accurate prescription for safe, quick relief of symptoms. Without testing it's a guessing game—and at the patient's expense.

Why I Wrote This Book

To tell you the truth, I wrote this book because I needed help myself. After the birth of my second baby, my postpartum depression was significant. I knew my "baby blues" were hormonal, but wanted more answers on how to treat it other than the usual birth control pills and Prozac. I wanted to feel well and enjoy my baby, but realized that I needed guidance beyond what I was getting. I also realized that most of my patients, at one point or another, had hormone-related problems, including depression, fatigue, weight gain, PMS (premenstrual syndrome), low sex drive, and early menopause symptoms.

After intensive independent study, numerous professional workshops and seminars led by prominent hormonal specialists, and working with more than ten thousand women in the area of hormonal imbalances, I developed a specialty practice focusing on diagnosing, testing, and treating female hormonal imbalances. I am continually in contact with women across the country through my own lectures, symposia, workshops, and meetings.

Women who seek my help typically have longstanding physical and emotional complaints that have been written off by medical providers as normal or genetic. I have grown to appreciate what women go through every day of their lives and have an increasing concern for the lack of women's hormonal care. I have gained a deep understanding of the intricacies of hormone testing, from conducting the tests to interpreting the results and following the patient to the point of balance.

I am passionate about helping women understand their options and realize that they do not need to live with symptoms of hormonal imbalance. I know that with careful testing and treatment, just about any woman's symptoms can be relieved safely and effectively.

How This Book Can Help

Use this book as a step-by-step guide to feeling better, getting on top of your perimenopausal symptoms, and entering menopause without wishing you could check out! It can serve as your map to achieving health and wellness and show you why it makes sense to find a medical provider who will test your hormone levels and take them into account when prescribing treatment. It will also explain in detail how exercising, managing stress, improving your diet, and taking supplements can help balance your hormones and make a new woman out of you.

The Hormone Survival Guide for Perimenopause offers solutions that you and your healthcare provider can adapt to your individual needs. It is laid out so that you may read chapters that specifically relate to your current symptoms or problems. Let it help you save precious time, money, and energy by giving you tools that will change your life—and most likely the lives of those around you. Good luck on your journey to wellness. The best is really yet to come!

Chapter 1

Why Hormonal Chaos?

IN THIS CHAPTER:

Current Medical Thinking About Hormones

The Hormone Roller Coaster

Hormones and Aging: Decline and Confusion

What Is Perimenopause and Why Do I Have to Go Through It?

There is no doubt that women's hormones are meant to operate in harmony. Hormone interactions have been compared to a ballet, a symphony—even barbershop harmonies. A stumble, a missed note, a voice off-key—all can trigger an unpleasant realization that something is not quite right. And so it is with hormonal balance. Complex hormone interactions and fluctuations throughout a typical menstrual cycle contribute in a major way to a woman's vibrancy and emotional and physical well-being. If hormones are out of sync, it's no secret. Most women, if asked the right questions, can describe how they feel and know intuitively when they are off-kilter. It is incredibly rewarding to help women understand their bodies, to know when systems are out of balance, and to guide them as hormonal problems begin to emerge during the aging process.

If you are experiencing unpleasant changes with age and are acutely aware that how you feel now is different from how you felt when you were younger, especially regarding your menstrual cycles, this book is for you; it will help you create harmony throughout your entire body.

You can be wonderfully healthy between thirty-five and fifty years of age if you are knowledgeable about what creates excellent hormonal balance and what to do if you find yourself out of sync. You may feel that your periodic upheavals are way out of control and worry that this is something much bigger than you can handle, but rest assured; if you know where the problem lies, and you take direct steps toward correction, relief is likely. Whether you are constantly dragging with fatigue, feeling irritable and headachy, or accumulating fat like never before, believe that you can move forward to create, maybe for the first time in your adult life, *hormonal balance.*

Current Medical Thinking About Hormones

In today's fast-paced medical world, doctors are pushed beyond their limits for time, resources, and patient management. Many are frustrated with packed schedules, sicker patients, and a burgeoning array of ever-changing medical tests and treatments. This is not a positive environment for a woman in her forties who is experiencing headaches, emotional lows, weight gain, and hot flashes. For many medical providers, responding to her complaints generally requires just a few minutes in the exam room. She is told that she is stressed out, has a poor diet loaded with too many calories, and, besides, she is probably depressed. More often than not, she is prescribed birth control pills and/or antidepressants and advised to reduce stress and clean up her diet. Wow, what a concept!

I find it completely crazy that if a woman complains of pain and numbness in her hand, she is quickly scheduled for myriad tests that may include X-rays, blood work, and sometimes even costly MRI (magnetic resonance imaging) scans. But if a woman in her forties reports to her medical provider that she is depressed, anxious, tired, and not sleeping at night, the provider rarely orders diagnostic tests. Instead the woman is reassured that her symptoms are normal for her age and that perhaps with the use of expensive, risky medications—such as synthetic contraceptives, antidepressants, antianxiety agents, and sleeping pills—her problems will disappear.

I am not sure how we ever got to the point in medicine where we cannot look logically at the female cycle and, with current understanding about the decline and fluctuation of women's hormones with age, simply explore, test, educate, and treat them. Instead, underlying hormone-related symptoms are masked—but not corrected—with medicines that most women do not need.

The Hormone Roller Coaster

Over the past two decades, hormone-related problems have escalated. Fibroids, PMS, endometriosis, infertility, breast cancer, cystic breasts, polycystic ovarian syndrome, and dramatic perimenopausal problems are more prevalent and are starting much earlier in women's lives.

It is at once fascinating and frightening to have witnessed firsthand these changes over the years and wonder why they appear to be on the rise. What is even more staggering is the number of hormone-related cancers. The 1997 "Report of Cancer" predicts that by 2015 the incidence of breast cancer will rise from 8.6 percent to 11.6 percent. The breast cancer risk has more than tripled in the past thirty years.

Premenstrual syndrome   Commonly known as *PMS*, premenstrual syndrome is another hormone-related affliction that is increasing dramatically. This syndrome plagues girls as young as ten, as well as women nearing menopause, at much higher rates than ever before. Not only are women experiencing more emotional changes with their cycles, but they are also suffering significant physical and mental side effects with their hormonal upheavals. I have seen in my own practice the growing number of women with disturbing monthly changes, women who typically did not have these problems in the past.

A survey conducted by the Women's Nutritional Advisory Service (WNAS) shows that 80 percent of women who suffer from PMS have had problems with depression, anxiety, and aggressive feelings; 52 percent of these women have contemplated suicide in the days leading up to the monthly period. The WNAS concludes that PMS is a twentieth-century phenomenon and a direct result of poor diet and increased stress. It is also interesting to note that this advisory team states that 90 percent of women who suffer from cyclic problems have complete resolution of symptoms within just four months when diet, exercise, and stress are managed.

Fibrocystic breast disease   Now afflicting approximately 25 percent of all women, those tiny, painful breast lumps that come and go with the cycle are closely related to estrogen and progesterone balance. Most often these lumps are benign, but women who suffer from them find it difficult to perform monthly breast self-exams. Fibrocystic breast disease also contributes significantly to an increase in the number of women needing additional mammography screens. When women's breasts are densely fibrocystic, identifying the normal tissue, versus a solid lesion, is difficult for the radiologist, frequently necessitating additional screening. Women suffer more discomfort; more radiation to sensitive breast tissue, probably unnecessarily; and certainly more anxiety! Other hormone-related female problems are on the rise as well.

Fibroids   These muscular growths within the uterine walls are estrogen driven. We know this because they often shrink in menopause and are not present in girls prior to menstruation. In my own practice, the number of women with fibroids is rapidly increasing. I routinely diagnose five to eight cases of fibroids weekly; just ten years ago, when my patient load was approximately the same, I saw perhaps two to three per month. An increase in the incidence of fibroids is most likely related to the escalating estrogen levels in women stemming from unnecessary use of medications, poor liver health, chronic stress, fat gain with age, obsessive intake of empty sugar-laden calories, and lack of exercise. All of these negative influences contribute to a poor hormonal environment that can promote estrogen dominance and fibroid growth. Unfortunately, stress, lifestyle behaviors, and the uniqueness of each woman make hormone-related conditions extremely difficult to research. As a result, there are no definitive studies that demonstrate with cold, hard facts some of the correlations that we know to be true in our medical practices.

Hormones and Aging: Decline and Confusion

Female hormones change dramatically with age. Their rise and fall may cause significant symptoms in some women, whereas others seem to skate through without any notable discomfort. What's normal for one woman may bear scant resemblance to what's normal for her best friend. So getting our arms around exactly what is happening—or what exactly we can *expect* to happen—can be confounding. The important thing to note is what's normal for one woman may not be normal for another.

The hormones we are most concerned with in this book are estrogen, progesterone, and testosterone. It is important to understand the roles these three hormones play in the female body and what happens when they are out

> **Hormone Levels Decline with Age**
>
> **Estrogen:** A 30 percent drop occurs by age fifty, with significant fluctuations during the forties and often the early fifties. In the first five years of menopause, the level declines sharply.
>
> **Progesterone:** A 75 percent loss occurs from age thirty-five to fifty and continues to decline.
>
> **Testosterone:** A 50 percent loss occurs from age twenty-five to fifty, and another 50 percent loss takes place by age eighty.

Figure 1-1   The decline of hormones with age

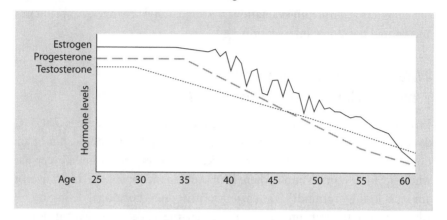

of balance. I offer my patients the metaphor of a symphony orchestra: When all members are playing in harmony, the sound and the effect are beautiful; when our hormones are playing from the same score, we can waltz through life. But when their notes are off-key, we begin to lurch and stagger. Too much estrogen and not enough progesterone and testosterone can make for some sour notes, and a true cacophony can be created by severe imbalance.

Figure 1-1 illustrates the steady decline of female hormones as women enter the perimenopausal years, thirty-five to fifty. Most women I see in my practice do not realize how hormones decline with age and are mystified that they are feeling so very different from when they were younger.

For some of my patients, hormonal harmony has never been a reality. I see numerous women in their forties who have had menstrual problems, PMS, infertility, depression, and acne since they started their periods. They don't know what it's like to feel good. Other women in their late thirties may have always felt healthy, but the good times have come to a screeching halt. All of a sudden, they realize that they are worn out, irritable, and crying at things that didn't used to bother them. Worse yet, they have lost all interest in sex, when in the past they were insatiable.

It is crucial to start treatment before the bottom drops out. If I can work with a woman when she first begins to notice changes, the turnaround is often brief and she can go on her way. But if a woman comes to me after twenty years of hormonal havoc and has been on multiple medications and maybe has resorted to hysterectomy or other surgical interventions, the evaluation is more complex and the treatment more tedious. The good news is every woman can benefit from in-depth evaluations, testing, lifestyle changes, supplements, and natural hormonal intervention.

What Is Perimenopause and Why Do I Have to Go Through It?

Perimenopause is simply the years before menopause. Menopause is that one-day event when you get your very last natural period. Pretty simple, huh? I am not sure how we have made it so complicated. I work with women every day who say, "I just want to know where I am. Am I in menopause at thirty-five, or am I just losing my mind?" Some women insist on a "hormonal definition" of what category they fit into, and I always say the same thing: "What does it matter what you call it?" Not to sound unfeeling, but it is of little consequence what you label your particular stage in midlife unless you are trying to get pregnant and want to know for sure whether you are ovulating.

But think about it for just a moment: Your body is moving inevitably toward menopause, and when the time is right, you will have it. This biological event cannot be postponed. What we *can* do is change how we experience menopause and the years leading up to it. Basically, perimenopause is a matter of age. Women between thirty-five and fifty could be experiencing peri-menopausal symptoms, which may be constant or occurring intermittently. Age-related hormonal changes are taking place and will lead to the inevitable event: the final menstrual period.

As this fifteen-year stage begins, hormone levels fluctuate and periods begin to change. They may last a little longer or become farther apart than in the past. Some women experience mild headaches or insomnia in the days before the period begins. Other perimenopausal women are hanging on for dear life as they ride the hormonal roller coaster, plunging from the highest highs to the deepest lows in a matter of twenty-four hours. During these years each woman's response to hormone over- or underproduction is unique and dramatically affected by her lifestyle, environment, and genetic makeup.

As I see it, women experience perimenopause in one of three general ways:

1. There are women who are completely symptom-free until the day they stop having periods. Lucky them!

2. There are women who have mild hormonal dips and bumps, producing some symptoms before their periods or intermittently throughout their cycle. Their symptoms gradually increase with age and usually become significant before menopause.

3. There are women who have significant unpleasant symptoms, often on a daily basis. The days that are good are few, and there is a pronounced difference between good and bad days. Without intervention and life-style changes, the symptoms for these hard-hit women remain fairly constant until menopause.

Where do you fit in? Are you among the lucky women who skate through these years, or are you on the hormonal roller coaster? If you're like most women, you are experiencing a range of hormone-related symptoms from mild to horrendous. The following chapters will educate you about natural hormonal changes and offer detailed information about how to achieve balance and optimal health. Use this knowledge to journey successfully through some of the most important years of your life.

Chapter 2

Know Your Hormones in and out of Balance

IN THIS CHAPTER:

Perimenopause: The Change Before the Change

How Do Hormones Tip out of Balance?

The Hormonal Domino Effect

Hormonal Highs and Lows

Estrogen

Progesterone

Testosterone

Julianne was forty-three but felt fifty-five. Even though she had never had PMS, she was faltering now. She appeared in my office in tears, wondering why all of a sudden she'd gained 15 pounds, had night sweats and headaches before her period, and, perhaps worst of all, had lost all interest in sex. Depression and bouts of explosive anger had become unwelcome parts of her emotional life. She was exhausted and unhappy, and her self-image was in the toilet.

I had to tell Julianne, "Welcome to perimenopause!" I also reassured her that balancing her hormones was going to make a huge difference and that before long she would be feeling herself again. I said this with confidence because I have seen it time and again. When women between the ages of thirty-five and fifty experience significant changes in mood, weight, libido, and general well-being, unbalanced hormones are most often to blame. I have also seen that with careful testing and treatment, unbalanced hormones can most often be brought into equilibrium.

Sure enough, Julianne's estrogen levels were elevated, and her progesterone level was low. Progesterone has a lot to do with mood, and low levels are associated with depression, among other things. She was also deficient in DHEA, the energy and vitality hormone. Julianne started a regimen of bioidentical prescription progesterone, DHEA capsules, and a low-sugar diet, which increased her energy and reduced her body fat in short order. She noticed within one menstrual cycle that she had less cramping, a 75 percent reduction in PMS, no more night sweats, and better mood control. Three cycles later all of her hormone levels tested within normal range. Two years have passed since her original visit, and Julianne enjoys life free from perimenopausal or other hormonal problems. In addition, she has learned better nutrition—including proper use of supplements, stress control, and relaxation techniques—and the important role that regular exercise plays in physical and emotional well-being. She is also able to identify symptoms that could mean trouble and now takes care of them on her own.

Perimenopause: The Change Before the Change

As noted in chapter 1, you don't just wake up one day and find yourself in menopause. Changes leading to the final menstrual cycle—the *real* menopause—may sneak up so gradually that you hardly notice. Or they may career into your life like a nightmare roller coaster, taking you on a wild ride for which you never signed up. Women in perimenopause may be plagued by mood swings, depression, hot flashes, insomnia, weight gain, fatigue, and low sex drive, to name a few symptoms. Periods may get heavier or lighter, farther apart or closer together. Many women skip a period or two altogether and end up biting their nails over a pregnancy scare. The time frame for perimenopause can be as long as fifteen years, but for most women it begins in the forties and lasts for two to eight years.

Whether two years or fifteen, that's too long to feel badly, and most women seek solutions to the physical and emotional problems that surface during middle age. Let's be truthful: Age is relative. A friend once said, "If you think you're old now, wait five years." So a fifty-year-old woman thinks that a thirty-five year old is young. But the thirty-five year old, who is starting down the slope to forty and trying to adapt to being considered middle-aged, may be thinking, *Whoa! How did I get so old so fast?* In the meantime the fifty year old, who has come to terms, more or less, with middle age, is peeking around the corner at the next decade. Sixty is a terribly big number. Seventy? We don't even want to go there! Eighty and beyond? Unimaginable! The point is that life is continuous change, and we are always adapting. The sooner we accept change—and getting older—as inevitable and even desirable (who wants the alternative?), the sooner we can take full advantage of what each phase in life has to offer. Safely balancing or replenishing hormones can help women enjoy life no matter what their age.

Many women in the perimenopausal years are growing spiritually and emotionally. They are transitioning from the demands of caring for young children or the stress of starting a career to a new phase, where they are exploring where they're going and how they want to get there—that is, unless they are hobbled by depression, PMS, weight gain, exhaustion, and other perimenopausal symptoms that get in the way of their dreams.

Ideally, perimenopausal women are in a place where they can implement dietary changes, self-help measures, and other lifestyle improvements to relieve their symptoms. Two decades ago—and some would say even today—most women endured these symptoms and believed doctors who told them, "It's all in your head" or "This is just the way it is for women." Well, most women aren't taking it anymore. They are asking questions that demand solutions: *What can I do about my depression? What about my in-the-pits sex drive, my memory lapses, and my weight gain? What can I do to feel good again?*

I am so glad to tell patients that answers exist and are within reach of just about every woman. In the following chapters, I provide simple solutions and, in some cases, quick fixes to common problems. You too can gain control of your hormonal balance and, like Julianne, be able to breeze through the years leading to menopause!

How Do Hormones Tip out of Balance?

Let's start with the basics. Hormones are essential to life. They are chemical connectors to the brain, muscles, sex organs, and virtually every part of the body. If you were suddenly without the intricate communication conducted via hormones, you would quickly die. As it is, a missed message, a broken connection, or unclear communication from one hormone to another can cause an imbalance, upsetting the whole shebang. Pretty soon you're walking around wondering what hit you upside the head.

An estimated 50 to 70 million women are in perimenopause today. As early as a woman's mid-thirties, a drop in estrogen or progesterone, or a break in the ovulation (releasing an egg) cycle, can cause the domino effect of mood instability, weight gain, skin problems, and many other changes. Despite the fact that just about every woman knows she will eventually experience menopause, these changes can come as unpleasant surprises. Unfortunately, medical providers are often too rushed to fill her in on what's happening with her biochemistry. Here's a quick explanation.

The female hormone cycle, while extremely intricate, provides most women with hundreds of easy, normal menstrual cycles. Then she enters the perimenopausal years, and things begin to change. Ovulation occurs approximately fourteen days after the first day of the previous period. From the time a woman ovulates until her next period begins, the hormonal system gives feedback as to whether the woman is pregnant. If not, estrogen and progesterone levels start to decline, which brings on another period. During perimenopause, the drops in estrogen and progesterone are significantly steeper, creating mood swings and physical symptoms not present in earlier years.

Physical and emotional problems are aggravated if her diet is heavy in sugar and worthless white-flour carbohydrates, or if relentless stress is not controlled. A history of chronic health problems can leave a woman vulnerable to a hormonal crisis. Whatever the cause, hormonal imbalances are not uncommon. The good news is that you and your hormones can be brought back into balance.

The Hormonal Domino Effect

The hormonal domino effect begins with fluctuating progesterone levels. Progesterone, desperately needed for emotional and physical balance, can vacillate under the influence of diet, stress, and vitamin and nutrient intake. When progesterone dips, estrogen levels rise to compensate. When we have too much estrogen, a condition known as *estrogen dominance,* bad things begin to occur; these include acne, bloating, weight gain, fibrocystic breasts, fibroid uterine tumors, unstable emotions, and irritability. Menstrual irregularities such as heavy periods, cramping, or missed periods can also result. It usually isn't just one thing that causes a hormonal imbalance. The foods that we eat—primarily those high in sugar or that turn into sugar quickly upon entering our mouths, such as breads, pastas, crackers, and cereals—can raise insulin, the fat-storage hormone. This rise in insulin can trigger changes in the natural hormone cycle, causing fatigue, depression, weight gain, and irregular periods.

It has been my experience that medications such as antidepressants, steroids, antibiotics, and inhalers can also disrupt the hormone cycle. This is not surprising when you consider that these medicines put an additional load on the liver, which at the same time is trying to maintain hormonal balance by metabolizing and excreting hormones.

And then there's stress—perhaps the most insidious trigger for hormonal flip-flops. When you're tense, apprehensive, and emotionally overloaded, your hormones can be all over the map. If you doubt the power of stress over your well-being, try living through a period of prolonged, unrelenting stress, such as a divorce, a suddenly doubled workload, a wayward child or spouse, a cancer diagnosis, or any number of acutely distressing situations. After just a couple of weeks of such intense stress, most women experience mental, emotional, and physical effects; these can include menstrual irregularities, weight gain or loss, fragile mood, acne, and sleeplessness. Your periods may change, your breasts become sore, and maybe you have a sudden onset of PMS or headaches before your period. If you're lucky, these signs of hormonal change may be as temporary as the events that caused the imbalance in the first place.

No one is immune to the ill effects of prolonged stress. Maybe you know one of those lucky women who seem to bounce back no matter what: Their periods don't change; they don't gain weight; they don't get PMS. They just seem to plow right through it. Well, if stress continues to hit them on a daily basis, even they will burn out—and in no small way. No matter who you are, excessive chronic stress, medications used for other problems, genetics, weight gain, pregnancy, poor diet, or lack of exercise—all can set you up for a hormonal crash.

Hormonal Highs and Lows

So something happens, whether it's stress, diet, or medications—or a genetic predisposition—and your hormones either revert to a normal state or they don't. It depends on how healthy you are to begin with. The key is to take care of yourself so you're not as susceptible to inevitable hormone fluctuations. Even though much of what happens in life is beyond your power, you *can* control what you eat, how much you exercise, and whether you use vitamin and herbal supplements.

Let's take a look at the female sex hormones. We'll find out what they do, and I'll share my experience in testing and treating their imbalances.

Estrogen

Estrogen is what makes women feminine. It affects our sex organs and shapes our hips and breasts—and even our vocal cords. Estrogen transforms girls into women. Because of estrogen, our skin glows, our breasts are full, and we feel sensual. Our eyes sparkle because of the moisture estrogen brings to them.

Estrogen lubricates the vagina and prepares the womb during the menstrual cycle for implantation of the egg. There are hundreds of estrogen receptors throughout the body. This amazing hormone maintains blood-sugar levels and protects against osteoporosis, heart disease, Alzheimer's disease, colon cancer, Parkinson's disease, incontinence, and tooth loss. Estrogen receptors are also plentiful in the brain, where they help the brain cells make connections, allowing our mind to stay sharp, our memory to be sound, and our emotions to remain stable.

Three types of estrogen are produced by the ovaries and, to a lesser extent, by the adrenal glands. *Estradiol* is the most potent estrogen and is the one in greatest evidence in premenopausal women. *Estrone* is the dominant estrogen after menopause and is associated with fat storage. *Estriol* is the weakest form and is at its highest levels during pregnancy.

Estrogen fluctuates throughout the normal monthly cycle and is most abundant around ovulation, which is usually halfway between the end of one period and the beginning of the next. Note in figure 2-1 how estrogen starts out fairly low the first day of your period, but then rises at ovulation, peaking at around day 12. Estrogen then drops off gradually before the next period begins.

Estrogen levels begin fluctuating by age thirty-five, primarily because women ovulate less as they age. Without ovulation, progesterone levels drop significantly, often causing an estrogen spike to compensate. Instead of a gradual decline of estrogen prior to their periods, some women experience abrupt highs and lows, causing hot flashes, night sweats, insomnia, fatigue, and low sex drive

Figure 2-1   Normal estrogen levels during the month (as indicated by estradiol)

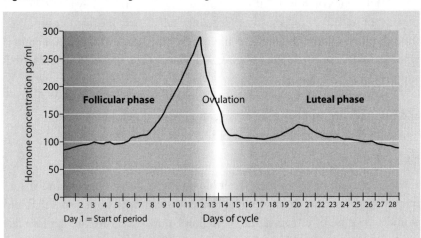

Figure 2-2   Effects of high and low estrogen

Too High	Too Low
Breasts tender and swollen	Hot flashes and/or night sweats
Bloating	Insomnia
Pounding headaches	Vaginal dryness
Weight gain—pooches around the middle	Decreased sexual sensation, lubrication, and drive
Volatile emotions	Mental fogginess
Uterine fibroids and/or fibrocystic breasts	Memory and concentration problems
Vaginal yeast infections	Depression and/or irritability
Unstable blood-sugar levels	Dry skin and brittle nails
Depression	Fatigue
Joint pain	Migraine headaches
Irritability	Frequent urination
Water retention	Flatulence, osteoporosis

(see figure 2-2). Significant estrogen peaks and dips can cause a woman to feel as though menopause is imminent. With estrogen levels high, and ovulation not occurring as often, progesterone levels dip. This particular imbalance between estrogen and progesterone is at the root of most perimenopausal symptoms. A major goal of hormone balancing is to restore progesterone to create equilibrium with estrogen.

What Is Estrogen Dominance?

Estrogen dominance, a term coined by Dr. John Lee, author of *What Your Doctor May Not Tell You About Premenopause,* refers to estrogen's predominating the hormone balance, is known by most hormonal experts to be a problem with many perimenopausal women. It describes a condition in which a woman's estrogen levels may be low, normal, or excessive, but she has little or no progesterone to balance the effects of estrogen on the body. Excess estrogen is associated with breast, ovarian, and uterine cancer as well as endometriosis (when fragments of the uterine lining are found in other parts of the body). We know that excessive estrogen causes uterine fibroids to grow larger and fibrocystic breasts to become denser.

In addition to naturally occurring hormone fluctuations, events and elements outside the body that can bring about estrogen dominance include the following.

Toxic stress   When a woman is under excessive stress, the adrenal glands send for energy backup in the form of cortisol. Cortisol production can eventually suppress progesterone production and increases estrogen levels.

Diet   Diets high in sugar and starch cause increased fat storage through the insulin hormone. Fat cells produce enzymes that increase estrogen levels in the blood. This stored excess estrogen can lead to weight gain, sore breasts, and heavy periods.

Birth control pills   The pill contains synthetic estrogen, which can cause nausea, weight gain, and other negative symptoms for women who already have high estrogen levels.

Sluggish liver   A healthy liver eliminates excessive circulating estrogen and sex hormone–binding globulin. Aging, caffeine, sugar, alcohol, and medications that impair liver function can reduce the elimination of excessive estrogen.

Illness   A viral infection can affect the functioning of the thyroid gland, and an imbalance of the thyroid hormones can negatively influence progesterone and estrogen production.

Xenohormones   Somehow many synthetic chemicals in today's environment are able to communicate with cells in a pattern almost exactly like that of estrogen. They can also suppress the immune system. The prefix *xeno* means "foreign." So a *xenohormone* is an element from outside the human body that performs a hormonelike communication inside the body. Research published in 2000 in the *Archives of Pediatrics and Adolescent Medicine* shows that both boys and girls are reaching puberty earlier. Researchers speculate that poor diet plays a role, as well as exposure to environmental chemicals that affect hormone function. Xenohormones have also been implicated in breast cancer development and many other illnesses.

Hysterectomy/oophorectomy   When a woman's uterus and ovaries are removed, progesterone production virtually stops, which can create estrogen dominance and result in depression, fatigue, weight gain, and loss of sex drive.

Progesterone

Produced primarily by the ovaries, *progesterone* works with estrogen to prepare the uterus for conception. It thickens the uterine lining, essentially building a nest for the fertilized egg, and secretes nutrients that are important for the embryo. Progesterone works with estrogen, helping create a positive balance between the two hormones. One of its most important jobs is to prevent excess estrogen. Progesterone and estrogen give the best effect when they are balanced, which in turn creates fewer bleeding problems and more equilibrium going into menopause.

Progesterone makes its monthly surge in the second half of the menstrual cycle, just opposite the surge of estrogen in the first half. As you can see in figure 2-3, the progesterone level stays fairly low and constant in the first half of the cycle. Following ovulation it surges and peaks at about day 18. The progesterone level gradually subsides until day 28, just in time for the next period to begin.

Progesterone, or the lack thereof, begins to wreak havoc for women when the levels in the second half of the cycle are not prominent. Progesterone is the mood hormone, and during the two weeks leading up to the period, it is extremely important to maintain normal to high levels. A low progesterone level paves the way for estrogen dominance to create PMS symptoms and emotional imbalance. The more infrequently a woman ovulates, the less progesterone she produces.

Figure 2-3   Normal progesterone levels during the month

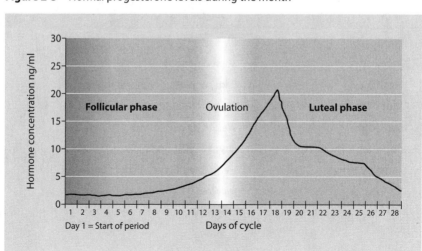

The Benefits of Progesterone

■ As a natural antidepressant, enhances moods and creates a calming effect

■ Provides healthiness to skin, hair, and nails and helps prevent hair loss

■ Regulates fluid balance, acting like a natural diuretic

■ Helps burn fat for energy and provides necessary control for insulin regulation

■ Protects against endometrial cancer, fibrocystic breasts, and probably breast cancer

■ May protect against bone loss

■ Helps support the thyroid

■ Regulates body temperature

■ Controls monthly bleeding by normalizing blood clotting

■ In short, it affects nearly every part of your body

What Happens When Progesterone Levels Drop?

Most perimenopausal women eventually have low or low-normal progesterone levels. As a result, many experience early symptoms of menopause (see figure 2-4). With inadequate progesterone, women experience nervousness, depression, blue moods, irritability, mood swings, dry skin and hair, brittle nails, and erratic or heavy periods. Low progesterone is a known cause of PMS and postpartum depression.

Figure 2-4   Effects of high and low progesterone

Too High	Too Low
Fatigue	PMS
Dizziness	Missed periods
Weight gain	Rage, depression, and/or irritability
Light periods or absent periods	Breast tenderness
Headaches	Weight gain
Nipple tenderness	Dry skin, hair, and nails
Mental fogginess	Heavy bleeding and cramping with clotting
	Hair loss
	Infertility
	Insomnia

Testosterone

Testosterone is known as the forgotten hormone, especially in menopause, as many medical providers do not pay attention to the signs of its decline. Menopausal and perimenopausal women who have fatigue, muscle atrophy, weakness, low libido, and low sexual sensation often have low testosterone (see figure 2-5).

Present in both men and women, testosterone is produced in small amounts by the ovaries and the adrenal glands. Although men naturally make 50 percent more testosterone than women, it is a vital hormone that women rely on for energy, vitality, sex drive, and endurance. Testosterone does the following for the female system:

▶ Provides energy and vitality

▶ Builds muscle and helps promote muscle tone

▶ Regulates the sex drive and increases sexual sensation

▶ Helps with vaginal elasticity, lubrication, and muscle strength

▶ Strengthens bones and prevents osteoporosis

Whereas most perimenopausal women are short on testosterone, some have high levels. High testosterone levels can be caused by excessive stress, but the main disorder we look for is polycystic ovarian syndrome (PCOS), which can occur anytime during the menstruating years. If a woman has facial hair, weight gain, acne, and depression, it is likely that her testosterone levels are high and she may be suffering from PCOS. If you have had PCOS in the past,

Figure 2-5 Effects of high and low testosterone

Too High	Too Low
Increased facial hair	Fatigue and/or loss of zest for life
Irritability	Decreased libido
Nervousness	Decreased sexual sensation
Hair loss—premature alopecia	Decreased energy
Lack of periods	Osteoporosis
Aggression	Weight gain/fat gain
Acne on face and body	Loss of strength and/or endurance
Weight gain	Vaginal dryness

or if you struggle with what appears to be high levels of testosterone, you most likely will have excessive levels right up to menopause.

Stress can reduce testosterone in some women while increasing it in others. During perimenopause, when ovulation becomes irregular and progesterone decreases, testosterone levels will likely decline at the same time. Women typically lose 50 percent of their testosterone between the ages of thirty-five and fifty-five.

Now that you have a better understanding of the three primary female hormones, we can move into the areas that are vital for restoring and maintaining their equilibrium. Understanding the highs and lows of female hormones can make the difference in ultimately balancing your system. It will also help you recognize problems as they arise either before or during treatment. Referring to figures 2-2, 2-4, and 2-5 to remain aware of hormonal highs and lows in the future will not only help guide your treatment plan, but will also provide a baseline for you that can be easily referred to as you assess and resolve your symptoms.

Chapter 3

Have Your Hormones Tested

IN THIS CHAPTER:

Why Test Your Hormones?

Timing Is Everything

Testing Options

Interpreting Lab Results

Working with Your Medical Provider

Long-term Hormonal Balance

When I told Shelly, age thirty-four, that she needed her hormone levels checked to get to the bottom of her troubling physical and emotional symptoms, she looked at me like I was crazy. Shelly had sprouted facial hair, was putting on a spare tire, had missed some periods, and was depressed—all signs of hormonal imbalance. But her doctor had discredited hormone testing, saying it couldn't be accurate because hormone levels in the blood fluctuate throughout the month. "Okay," I said. "We don't have to test; instead we will start guessing and maybe within a year or so we can figure it out through the process of elimination."

Shelly agreed to the tests, which revealed low levels of progesterone; high levels of estradiol, testosterone, and DHEA; and extremely high levels of insulin. I explained that the high testosterone and DHEA levels were associated with facial hair, and the high insulin levels accounted for the fat gain. The low progesterone attributed to her depression, and the high estrogen to her vile moods. When confronted with this news, she no longer looked at me like I was crazy, but as if I had known her all her life. Today, after treatment of her hormone deficiencies and excesses, she has no facial hair, wears size 10 pants—down from size 16—and has no signs of depression or fatigue. Her periods are back on track as well. What would we have done without the testing?

Why Test Your Hormones?

Hormone imbalances in women create a sorry spectrum of problems. Everything from weird periods to hot flashes, mood swings to weight gain, and libido doldrums to adult acne can be blamed on out-of-whack hormones. So doesn't it make sense to measure hormone levels to help explain symptoms, identify underlying problems, and accurately prescribe treatment?

For many women, especially those whose complaints have been dismissed by their doctors—or their significant others—with such comments as "You'll just have to live with it" or "It's all in your head," hormone testing and follow-up treatment can mean the difference between feeling good or going off the deep end. Without determining where a woman's hormones are compared with normal ranges, treatment is just a guessing game.

A woman on thyroid medicine is tested frequently to make sure she doesn't get a single microgram too much or too little. When a woman seeks help for hormone-related complaints, however, she's typically handed a prescription and booked back in a year, with no testing for before-and-after levels. If high estrogen levels can be a causative factor in the development of breast cancer—not to mention PMS, fibroids, and fatigue—and too little estrogen contributes to osteoporosis and other ills, why in the world isn't hormone testing routine?

Hormone testing is the best way to establish a baseline. Although the "normal" values may change for each patient—and not every woman fits within ranges that are somewhat artificial—testing still provides a guideline from which the treatment plan is created and tested against in the future. Fortunately, word about hormone testing is getting out, and women are asking for it. As a result, more and more medical providers are learning how to test and interpret hormone levels so that women can take control of their symptoms.

Each Woman Is Unique

Individuality is the name of the game with women's hormone testing and treatment. Even though women may have similar complaints, each has her own hormone profile, unique responses to treatment, and a singular lifestyle to which the program must be adapted. These variables make my job incredibly challenging, but also extremely rewarding. I have learned that the one-size-fits-all approach definitely does not apply, and I frequently remind patients that hormone balancing is not a science but an art. Women often come to my office with their lives broken into fragments. We work as partners to fit the pieces back together so that the woman eventually sees her physical and emotional sides merge as a harmonious whole. This is not instant medicine, but a process. Each patient must be keenly aware of what can cause hormonal disruption and realize that getting into a balanced state can take time.

Two perimenopausal patients who visited my office on the same day illustrate the need for individuality in treatment. Katie and Linda had nearly identical symptoms: depression, more pronounced before their periods; headaches; occasional insomnia; extreme irritability throughout the month; weight gain around the middle; and tender breasts before the period. After thoroughly evaluating their symptoms—which included a detailed history and a discussion about diet, stress, lifestyle, exercise, and family—I ordered serum (blood) tests for both in the later half of their menstrual cycles. The tests measure levels of estrogen, progesterone, free testosterone, FSH (follicle-stimulating hormone), DHEA-S, and a full thyroid panel and are ordered during the luteal phase of the cycle, which is at least 18 days after the first day of the previous period.

When their test results came back, I was not surprised to see that they were entirely different. Katie had a pronounced progesterone deficiency in the phase of her cycle when her body should be producing ample progesterone, and her estrogen level was very high. Her treatment plan included progesterone replacement with an action plan for reducing her excess estrogen. Linda, on the other hand, had a thyroid deficiency and low progesterone; her estrogen was at normal levels. Her treatment was thyroid replacement therapy with progesterone supplementation.

These two women with nearly identical symptoms illustrate the benefits of hormone testing to determine successful treatment plans. Without it the treatments probably would not have been so specific, and the outcomes most likely would not have been as good or as timely. Both patients went on to do extremely well and were relieved of nearly all their perimenopausal symptoms.

Bucking the Trend

When I first began ordering hormone tests for women, some physicians were critical. They maintained that testing is unreliable, expensive, and of no value whatsoever. It is interesting to note that the physicians making these remarks had received no additional training in hormone balancing, had never ordered a hormone panel, and, in some cases, refused to recognize that women should be treated individually. Of course I disagree and have hundreds of successful cases to back me up.

It is also of interest to note that both teaching universities that I have worked with in the past, which are well known for their medical research and development, not only utilize hormone testing, but now promote it. In a March 2003 study published by *Fertility and Sterility,* researchers found that serum hormone testing was of significant value when treating menopausal women with hormone therapy to help produce safe, effective dosing.

Testing patients whose symptoms are obviously cyclical or perimenopausal has made an enormous difference in women's healthcare. Some women are being validated for the first time; what they feel is *not* just in their heads after all, but real problems with effective solutions. The most impressive fact about serum hormone testing is that in most cases it correlates with the patient's symptoms. Many women who have had successful testing and hormonal intervention have been able to stop other medications prescribed to clear up problems stemming from hormonal imbalances.

The cost of hormone testing is a fraction of what many women pay physically, emotionally, and financially for the trial-and-error method of discovering which, if any, medications will relieve their symptoms. It is evident that with perimenopausal women, myriad complaints can be cleared up with a simple blood test to determine hormone levels, followed by a treatment plan to balance them. The cost of testing is a small price to pay for the peace of mind and the improved health that result.

Many experts in women's health agree that tests are reliable, accurate, cost-effective, and helpful in identifying the exact cause of a woman's symptoms. I am adamant that women should have access to both hormonal testing and the information they need to become advocates for their own hormonal care.

Dr. Christiane Northrup, author of the best-selling book *The Wisdom of Menopause* and a physician in the forefront of women's healthcare, is an advocate for hormone testing. She recommends that women's hormone levels be tested when perimenopausal symptoms begin. This means that if a woman is still menstruating, but is also noticing menopausal symptoms, testing can be ordered to establish a baseline and provide a guide if a hormone regimen is started later on.

The purpose of this chapter is to teach you how to ask your provider for what you need. Appendix A provides a list of laboratories used for testing and of national compounding pharmacies, any of which can provide a wealth of information regarding hormone testing and treatment.

Timing Is Everything

To obtain the most accurate results and determine whether you really need replacement therapy, testing at the correct time during the cycle is imperative. If you have regular menstrual cycles, the absolute best time to test is one week before the period begins. If your periods are irregular, count eighteen to twenty-one days after the first day of the previous period. This timing is important because you are most likely ovulating, the progesterone level is at its peak, and the circulating levels of estrogen and testosterone should be normal.

If you want to be tested for hormonal balance, ask your medical provider to order a serum (blood) panel of estradiol, progesterone, and testosterone one week before the period. On your own, you may order a saliva test for hormone levels. (See appendix A for a list of providers who will do the test by mail order.) Although many providers swear by saliva or urine testing, it has been my experience that serum testing is more useful in detecting hormone deficiencies and excesses and more valuable for ongoing comparisons. Many practitioners use saliva or urine testing (both of which do show deficiencies and excess levels) and find them helpful in monitoring their patients, and it works well in their practice. The important thing is to connect with a provider who does consistent testing with either of these methods.

If you are not having periods, or if you have had a hysterectomy but are experiencing menopausal symptoms, you may want to identify a time frame in which you feel worst and test then. If you cannot identify a worst time, testing at any time, or testing at two separate times two weeks apart, will help paint a definitive picture. Testing can also be done when you are feeling at your best to use as a comparison.

Testing Options

Hormone testing can be done through the serum (blood), saliva, or urine. These methods provide an effective, precise, and inexpensive means of monitoring the therapeutic response to hormone treatment or hormone deficiencies.

Serum (Blood) Testing

Serum testing is ordered by the medical provider and involves a simple blood draw in the doctor's office or at the lab. I regularly use serum testing to monitor the hormone levels in women who are experiencing symptoms at any age. Serum testing remains the worldwide gold standard for evaluating women's hormone levels and is routinely used by research organizations during studies of women's healthcare issues. Any medical laboratory can complete a serum test. Dr. Neal Rouzier has paved the way for medical providers to understand the importance and usefulness of serum testing in the area of hormone evaluation. He trained

Serum-Testing Specifics

1. Perform the test seven to ten days before your next expected period or at least eighteen to twenty days after the first day of your previous period. If your cycle is shorter than twenty-eight days, do the test seventeen to twenty days after the first day of your previous menstrual period.

2. Do not take hormones the day of the test. Try to take your last dose six to twelve hours prior to the test; if the test is done first thing in the morning, do not take your morning dose prior to testing. Resume your normal schedule following the blood draw.

3. When topical hormone preparations are used simultaneously with serum testing, you may find serum values lower than those seen with oral administration. This does not mean it is poorly absorbed.

4. Serum tests should be interpreted in relation to what day of the cycle the blood was collected. Days 1 to 13 of your cycle constitute the *follicular phase,* and days 14 to 28 make up the *luteal phase.* Knowing when the blood was drawn and what part of the cycle you were in will determine what your level should be at that specific time.

5. When unusually high values occur that do not correspond to how you are feeling, request a repeat sample. Occasionally, tests show a false high or low value. Any lab result that doesn't correlate with symptoms or that appears to be markedly off should be repeated for quality assurance.

6. If the value of progesterone is very high on days 18 to 21 of the cycle (indicating that you are ovulating), but you are experiencing PMS, headaches, or other cyclic problems, it may be due to a sharp decline in progesterone after the peak, leading to the onset of the period. Use of a bioidentical natural progesterone during the seven to ten days before the period can correct this problem, even when the progesterone level appears normal during testing.

7. There is no need to fast unless a thyroid panel is ordered.

8. Try to repeat the levels every three months until balance is achieved, then once annually. Serum testing can be repeated while using hormone treatment, but remember to not take your morning dose if the levels are drawn first thing in the morning. You are aiming to take the last dose of hormones at least six to twelve hours prior to the blood draw.

me as well as thousands of other medical providers across the nation, with the assistance and collaboration of MedQuest Pharmacy. MedQuest organizes regular training practicums, led by Dr. Rouzier, that are extremely useful for medical providers who want to design personal hormonal plans for women.

Although tests to measure hormone levels have been available for years, it is only recently that the sensitive radioimmunoassay tests have been available to clearly detect the levels in the blood. These tests also have standardized normal values, which make their interpretation more streamlined. Laboratories have set standards for women's hormone levels based on normal cyclic ranges that extend from the perimenopausal period into the menopausal time frame. The standards eliminate guesswork and make pinpointing problems much easier. To determine if the level is in the normal range, it is of utmost importance that the medical provider interpreting the test results knows where the patient is in her cycle. The optimal levels of both estrogen and progesterone change throughout the month, so it is imperative to know when the test was done in relation to the cycle.

Serum testing is convenient, timely, accurate, and covered by most insurers. More and more medical providers are ordering hormone testing for women during the transitional years of perimenopause. This may be due to the ongoing medical controversies over hormone replacement therapy; women are beginning to ask for testing so that they supplement with just the right amount. It also may be because medical providers realize the prudence of documenting a woman's need for supplementation before prescribing HRT.

Patients who request hormone testing may be told that, because levels fluctuate throughout the cycle, testing is not accurate or helpful. If you are fed this line, don't swallow it. Hormone researchers routinely use serum testing to identify levels in women before and during treatment. All research studies that investigate the effects of estrogen and other hormones use blood testing to measure effects throughout the study period. Hormone consultants around the world rely on hormone testing to conduct their evaluations, and such teaching schools as Oregon Health & Science University conduct seminars to educate medical providers on the importance of hormone testing.

The information that has come to light through measuring my patients' hormone levels has been crucial in everything from alleviating PMS to deterring the agonizing effects of depression and chronic fatigue syndrome. It has made the difference in preventing suicide, alleviating excruciating headaches, and curtailing weight gain. In my practice it would be difficult to do meaningful work with women and their hormonal imbalances without hormone testing.

Saliva Testing

This method requires that a small amount of saliva be collected in a tube for evaluation. Saliva testing can be done at a specific time during the menstrual cycle, or multiple samples can be taken throughout the month to evaluate the entire cycle. Saliva contains an abundant amount of free-circulating hormones and is an excellent indicator of progesterone levels. It is the only test that can map your personal cycle and demonstrate the rise and fall of estrogen and progesterone throughout the month. Included in the panel for female balance is an evaluation of testosterone and DHEA levels.

Saliva testing can be done in a one-sample fashion, looking at single measurements of estrogen, progesterone, and testosterone. Taking nine to eleven samples over the course of one full twenty-eight-day menstrual cycle is also effective. This can be helpful for women who have symptoms all over the calendar and do not know what time of the month is worst. This is the only test available that actually shows the female cyclic changes throughout the month. It is also particularly helpful in identifying ovulation timing and whether estrogen and progesterone are balanced throughout the cycle.

The saliva test can be ordered through your medical provider, or you can refer to appendix A to choose a laboratory from which to order a test. These laboratories help with the interpretation and will identify any abnormal values that will help pave the way for treatment by your medical provider.

Urine Testing

Although most doctors do not currently offer urine testing of hormones, it is still a viable option and is very accurate at showing the levels of hormones in the system. Urine testing requires that you collect your entire urine output over a twenty-four-hour period. It also requires that you use a lab equipped to analyze urine specimens for hormone testing. The advantage of the urine test is that it provides a full daily picture of your hormone levels, instead of a measure of a discrete point in time that serum offers. The urine testing for some will reveal deficiencies or hormonal excess that other tests may fail to pick up. The downside to this type of testing is finding a lab that is able to process the sample (see appendix A) and the inconvenience of a twenty-four-hour collection.

Interpreting Lab Results

In my clinical experience, I've found that women typically have their best energy and mood stabilization with optimal sleep patterns when serum (blood) levels

Saliva-Testing Specifics

1. Select the right test for you. If you are menstruating and the cycles occur once every twenty-one to forty-two days, a full saliva panel may be the best way to evaluate any hormonal changes. Saliva testing requires that you take multiple samples throughout the month and, once they are all collected, send them in for evaluation. If your cycles are nonexistent, if your periods are irregular, or if you've had a hysterectomy, a single sample or two samples done two weeks apart may be helpful in identifying abnormal ranges of hormones.

2. Saliva testing evaluates the free levels of hormones, which is a smaller representation of the total hormones in the body. This is important to know because a test showing low levels represents a fairly significant finding; it will most likely mean that you will be more symptomatic. Saliva contains a smaller proportion of hormones than is found in blood, so when the levels are low, they are *really* low.

3. Be cautious with saliva testing while using topical hormones: A lab must take this into account when providing results, or unusually high levels could occur.

4. If sublingual (under-the-tongue) preparations of hormones are used, the accuracy of saliva testing is compromised due to the retention of hormones in the oral mucosa.

5. If you are already using progesterone creams or sublingual preparations, the saliva tests in some circumstances will show false high levels and will be difficult to interpret. Consider using serum testing for follow-up, or again utilize a saliva lab that takes into account that you are on the topical hormone preparations.

6. If collecting a full saliva panel (over a twenty-eight-day cycle), as opposed to a single sample, collect exactly as directed. Freeze the samples and accurately document the day of your cycle on each collection. It would be additionally helpful to document your symptoms throughout the month to compare with the results.

7. If you are in your thirties or forties and experiencing perimenopausal symptoms, but would like to achieve pregnancy, the full saliva panel will be more useful than the one-sample test. This will help determine the timing of ovulation and any deficiencies in progesterone in the second half of the cycle that could prevent you from becoming pregnant.

8. If a serum test failed to explain your symptoms, do a full saliva panel, which incorporates multiple samples over the entire month.

9. If you are missing periods, a one-sample test is adequate if done at least eighteen days after the start of your last menstrual period.

10. Testing can be self-ordered at a number of laboratories (see appendix A). Your medical provider can also order a saliva test. Some testing facilities provide consultation on test results as well as treatment guidelines.

of estradiol are above 90 picograms per milliliter (pg/ml). This is assuming that the testing has been done in the week before the period. The level should not exceed 250 pg/ml, as this may indicate signs of estrogen dominance. When the level is above 90 pg/ml, women will have fewer perimenopausal symptoms. These blood levels are very helpful in determining the cause of the symptoms. A 1998 study published in the *American Journal of Obstetrics and Gynecology* showed that after a woman goes through menopause, she will most likely suffer from menopausal symptoms if the serum estradiol level falls below 50 pg/ml. Research is now beginning to show that testing is important in achieving ideal levels with the treatment.

The cyclical phases of estradiol and progesterone are shown in figure 3-1, and their rise and fall show distinct patterns. As you can see, estradiol peaks around midcycle, and progesterone peaks about seven to ten days before the period begins. If you test seven to ten days before the period, the levels of progesterone should be at least in the midrange to high end of normal. If the progesterone level is ordered during this time and returns at 1.2 ng/ml, which is below normal, supplementation with progesterone could be helpful. Even if the progesterone level is 3.0 (which is at the low end of normal), and perimenopausal symptoms are present, using progesterone to raise the level to the midrange could be beneficial in alleviating mood swings, bloating, cyclic weight gain, hot flashes, and insomnia (see figure 2.4).

Estradiol

> Normal range for estradiol (done seven to ten days before the period is to begin) is 80 to 240 picograms per milliliter (pg/ml).

Estradiol is the most potent of the three estrogen hormones, estradiol, estrone, and estriol. Together they are essential for the healthy functioning of the reproductive system and for breast development. The estradiol level fluctuates less in the second half of the cycle, and levels should decline toward the lower end of normal limits closer to the period (see figure 3-1). If the normal range for estradiol seven to ten days before the period is 80 to 240 pg/ml, the closer one gets to the onset of the period, the lower the number should be. If the test were done five days before the period and the level returned as 200 pg/ml, estrogen dominance would be the diagnosis (because the estradiol level is on the high end of normal), and symptoms could include fibrocystic breasts, heavy periods, and depression. High estradiol levels are nearly always associated with low levels of progesterone, and supplementing with progesterone will bring the ratio of progesterone to estradiol into a more normal range.

Figure 3-1 The cyclical phases of estradiol and progesterone

Estradiol

Hormone concentration pg/ml

Follicular phase | Ovulation | Luteal phase

Day 1 = Start of period | Days of cycle

Progesterone

Hormone concentration ng/ml

Follicular phase | Ovulation | Luteal phase

Days of cycle

Normal and optimal hormone ranges
For women still menstruating; samples taken within three to twelve days before the period.

Hormone	Normal Range	Optimal Range	Comments
Estradiol	80–240 pg/ml	90–120 pg/ml	The closer you are to your period, the lower the number should be, but not below 80.
Progesterone	2.0–17.0 ng/ml	5.0–17.0 ng/ml	The closer you are to your period, the lower the number should be, but not below 2.0. Levels peak around day 18 of the cycle.
Testosterone	2.2–8.0 ng/dl	3.0–5.0 ng/dl	Testosterone remains fairly stable throughout the month; testing should be done in the morning if possible. Most women experience an optimal libido around 4.0.

If the test for estradiol is drawn ten days before the period and the level returns at 80 pg/ml, you know the level is too low, even though it is still in the "normal" range. If you know the predictable rise and fall of estradiol within a cycle (see figure 3-1) and know which day in the cycle the woman was tested, even if her estradiol level is "normal" it may not be "optimal" according to where she should be in the cycle range. The important thing is to first be sure that testing occurs during the right part of the cycle and to interpret the test results accordingly. If a woman has symptoms associated with the low or high levels indicated, supplementation with hormones or other modalities can be advantageous.

Testosterone

> Normal range for testosterone for a thirty- to fifty-year-old
> woman is 2.2 to 8.0 nanograms per deciliter (ng/dl).

Testosterone levels are more constant and when measured should be closer to the midrange of normal. Women typically experience their most optimal energy and libido when the free-testosterone level is between 3.0 and 6.0 ng/dl. The "free" level of testosterone should always be the first choice when testing the serum levels, but if a "total testosterone" were ordered, the optimal range should be between 40 and 60 ng/dl. If the normal range for testosterone is 2.2 to 8.0 and a level for a thirty-year-old woman is around 2.2, she may experience reduced libido and low energy. Even though 2.2 is just within the normal range, this level would be considered too low for her to feel her best. On the other hand, if the level returned at 9.0 ng/dl and the woman is experiencing acne, weight gain, and excessive body hair, measures should be taken to reduce the testosterone level. (See chapter 2 for more about testosterone.)

Again, this is not a perfect science, and what works for one woman may not be effective for another. Achieving optimal hormonal balance takes investigation and time on the part of both the patient and her medical provider.

Working with Your Medical Provider

The good news is that a growing number of healthcare providers are now familiar with bioidentical hormones and hormone-testing options and are working with pharmacists who specialize in compounding individualized prescriptions. The bad news is that your doctor may not be one of them. If your medical provider does not know about testing or the use of natural hormones, your best bet is to seek out a provider who does, if only for your gynecological care and/or for hormone testing and treatment. It is a good idea to speak with a compounding pharmacy in your area about obtaining a list of medical providers who are proficient in testing (see appendix A for a list of compounding pharmacies).

Self-treating with herbs, over-the-counter remedies, or nonprescription hormone creams may be helpful, but most women need testing and evaluation from a trained hormonal specialist. Careful monitoring once treatment is started is as important as arriving at a diagnosis. The relationships among hormones are extremely intricate and complex. Treating one hormone can and will affect the balance of the others, which makes it imperative that the medical provider be knowledgeable about treating hormonal imbalances without causing an excess in any one hormone.

Although this chapter provides specific guidelines for hormone testing and interpretation, I am not suggesting that you take on your own medical care—hormonal balance is far too intricate to learn from reading one book. My aim is to equip readers with the basic knowledge that will help them to get the hormonal care they need. Although the number of practitioners who recognize the benefits of hormone testing and treatment with bioidentical hormones is growing, it is still news to many.

Women who know what they want are more likely to get the best care. You have the power and the right to request the exact test you want, and you should request a copy of the results so that you may check to see that your prescribed treatment is on track with your hormone levels. This helps to make you an active partner in your care rather than a passive observer. Just remember that interpreting the test results and ordering the appropriate hormonal balance is as important as ordering the tests in the first place. Perimenopausal symptoms can occur sporadically, which can make testing difficult. But with the appropriate testing and interpretation, a woman's relief can be significant.

Long-term Hormonal Balance

Lifestyle changes, such as excessive prolonged stress, poor diet, lack of activity, and the use of supplements or medications can disrupt the hormone balance that was so carefully achieved. The remaining chapters will help you steer clear of pitfalls and lead you toward life changes to help you achieve and maintain total wellness.

Chapter 4

Use Hormones to Treat Hormone Problems

IN THIS CHAPTER:

Natural Versus Synthetic Hormones

Individualizing Hormone Treatment

How to Use Progesterone

Estrogen Therapy in Perimenopause

What About Testosterone?

Moving Forward with Hormonal Balance

When she was just twenty-eight, Michelle was told she was in premature menopause. She had hoped to have children and had endured years of infertility testing, surgeries, and treatment, only to find out that the final diagnosis was "premature ovarian failure," in which hormones were not being produced. Michelle's periods had ceased, and she was suffering from hot flashes, vaginal dryness, night sweats, and mild depression; she had given up on her dreams of having a baby. Michelle then made an appointment with my office to discuss menopausal testing, counseling, and treatment.

After exploring possible causes of Michelle's lack of periods and her multiple menopausal symptoms, I ordered a full hormone profile, which included blood levels of estrogen, progesterone, testosterone, thyroid, and DHEA. The tests showed low levels of thyroid, progesterone, and testosterone and borderline low levels of estrogen. Michele started on progesterone, thyroid, and testosterone. (Estrogen was held to begin later.) Despite her diagnosis of premature menopause and ovarian failure, Michele began having regular periods within three months and was pregnant without any infertility treatment within six. She had repeat labs once prior to getting pregnant, which showed excellent hormonal balance.

Michelle is now the proud, happy mother of a baby girl and has regular menstrual cycles without taking hormone medication. She speaks to many women who are experiencing menopause or perimenopausal symptoms about the importance of testing and intervention. She tells women, as do I, that each woman has her own individual hormone profile, and when out-of-whack hormones are brought into balance, the outcomes can be nothing short of amazing.

Natural Versus Synthetic Hormones

Replenishing hormones and creating balance in the midst of hormonal upheaval can transform a woman's life. Even if that sounds like an outrageous claim, it isn't. Time and again I've seen women who have been lower than grass on a putting green one moment and higher than a weather balloon the next brought into equilibrium by the careful use of natural hormones. *Natural hormones* are hormones in their purest form—bioidentical in molecular structure to those made by the human body. They are made from plant material (either wild yam or soy), have the same effect as the body's own hormones, and do not interfere with the body's own hormone production. Used with care, they can have an excellent effect and resolve most hormone-related symptoms.

We are hearing a great deal today about natural hormones, and women's interest about choices outside what modern medicine has set before them is heightened. Unfortunately, women are often at the mercy of the commercial mass media, not to mention medical providers who have been influenced by pharmaceutical manufacturers' sales representatives. Information disseminated by the drug sales force is obviously profit-driven, and articles about hormone replacement in the popular media often present conflicting information.

A couple of myths have been established. The first is that if we don't use synthetic hormones, we will grow old before our time; second, if we *do* use them, we will surely get breast cancer and/or heart disease. Both of these claims are obviously untrue. Exploring the Internet can also be overwhelming and confusing. News reports are ever changing and often conflicting, and an aura of fear, insecurity, and misinformation surrounds hormone use.

In my experience, women feel much better about their decision to use a hormone prescription after a thorough hormonal screening and evaluation has pinpointed their exact deficiency or excess—and when they understand what they are taking. Hormone testing makes treating a hormonal imbalance much more precise and helps the patient become involved in her own care and decision-making. Additionally, it reinforces the need for each woman to be treated as a unique being.

The hormones that most medical providers prescribe are synthetic products manufactured in a lab—molecules that mimic the effects of the natural hormones produced by the human body. Synthetic hormones often differ in molecular structure from those produced by the body and therefore are not an exact match. The analogy I use with my patients is a key fitting into a keyhole: The key (the hormone) is either an exact fit and will open the door, or it is slightly different and will open it only with jamming, filing, or other fiddling.

Most synthetic estrogen is chemically based. *Medroxyprogesterone acetate,* the most commonly prescribe progestin, is synthetically derived, as is *methyltestosterone,* a commonly prescribed testosterone. These formulations are chemically based compounds that are similar but not identical to that produced by the human body. Because they do not have identical molecular structures, however, there are bound to be doors they can't open.

Does your body know the difference between natural progesterone that is identical in structure to the human body's and synthetic progesterone that is chemically based and not even close to human progesterone? In my opinion, *yes.* Although the human body's intuitiveness is still beyond the grasp of the human mind, it is safe to say that the cascade of effects brought about by the release of estrogen into the body is not quite the same when the estrogen is synthetically altered to mimic the effects of your body's own estrogen.

The word *natural* itself can be confusing. I find that some of my new patients believe that *natural* equates with over-the-counter herbs and vitamins and other nonprescription remedies that are seen as less effective than prescription drugs manufactured by pharmaceutical companies. *Not true!* Natural hormones, which have sparked considerable interest in recent years, are made primarily from soybeans and wild yams and are processed to create molecules identical to hormones made by the female body. Powerful and effective, they contain unique compounds that enable compounding pharmacies to formulate plant-based hormone substitutes. This exact replication allows the female body to recognize the hormone as its own and use it to its full potential. So *natural,* for our purposes, does not refer to the hormones' plant-based origins, but to the fact that these hormones function in exactly the same way as your own hormones.

My experience with natural hormones versus synthetics is that they provide more-complete correction of symptoms with fewer side effects. It appears that medicine may have come full circle in the area of hormones, as they originally were formulated and extracted from plants and have been in existence for more than fifty years.

Individualizing Hormone Treatment

Recognizing and respecting individuality is the absolute most important aspect of treating women for hormone-related problems. Each has a unique symptom profile and hormone test results, so the one-size-fits-all approach is inexact and inappropriate. Each woman experiences menstruation, pregnancy, perimenopause, and menopause differently, and throwing similar-dose birth control pills or synthetic estrogen at her to relieve perimenopausal symptoms is totally wrong. This generalization and narrow evaluation of unique hormonal systems is a disservice to many women.

Two women with different hormone test results but similar symptoms require individualized treatment plans. Each requires specific and unique adjustments, as her body utilizes the hormones at different rates. Some women metabolize hormones quickly and require smaller doses, whereas others require larger doses and longer treatment periods. Such highly individualized treatment is not possible without ongoing testing and close contact with the patient until her difficulty is resolved. Doctor and patient must establish a high level of open communication and trust, and patient education and involvement in treatment is essential. Consulting or involving a trained compounding pharmacist is extremely helpful in bridging the gap between the patient and the medical practitioner, and working toward a triad relationship with each person participating in the care can facilitate an excellent outcome. You may have already figured out that this approach is often unpopular in today's fast-paced medical practices.

If you use any hormone to create a more positive balance in your cycle, the result will be unique to you and different from that of your mother, sister, friend, or co-worker. Hormone dosing recommendations are based on a woman's personal profile, symptoms, risk factors, and medication history. I also base dosages on my experience in treating thousands of patients and in knowing how women's reactions to hormones can differ. As you begin any treatment with natural hormones, or even with some alternative complementary supplements suggested later in the book, you will observe your body's response.

Soon you will have a heightened awareness of how you are feeling and the necessary adjustments you should make.

As you go through the perimenopausal years, your hormonal needs will change, and periodic testing and adjustments will be needed. Constant changes are not roadblocks to treatment or testing, as some medical professionals have stated, but a reality that must be acknowledged by both the patient and the medical provider. The fact that women's hormones are in constant flux does not mean that hormonal balance cannot be achieved or that replenishing deficiencies is not necessary. What it *does* mean is that medical professionals must take the time and energy to get to know their patients' unique hormone profiles. Routine therapy must include gaining an understanding of a woman's unique symptoms and relieving them with individualized treatment. It isn't all up to the medical provider, however. A woman who chooses to be treated for hormonal imbalances must take care to understand her personal medical profile and work closely with her provider to make adjustments when necessary.

How to Use Progesterone

Insufficient progesterone is the most common hormone deficiency I see in perimenopausal women. As you learned in chapter 3, the normal range for progesterone is broad. Testing is best done within seven to ten days before the period begins. The treatment goal is to make sure that the progesterone level is above 5.0 ng/ml at its peak (day 21 of the cycle). Some women do not feel in control of their symptoms unless the level is at 10 to 15 ng/ml and may need to be on the upper end of normal limits to obtain the optimal effect.

Progesterone Versus Synthetic Progesterone (Progestin)

There are some important differences between bioidentical, natural progesterone and synthetic progesterone, or *progestin.* The substance known pharmaceutically as *Provera (medroxyprogesterone acetate),* or another one known as *norethindrone acetate,* can have significant side effects and rarely helps perimenopausal women with progesterone-deficiency symptoms. This is important to know, as many medical providers are familiar with the negative effects of progestins, but are not familiar with the positive mood-balancing effects of bioidentical, plant-based progesterone; they are as different as aspirin and Tylenol. When testing serum progesterone levels, the only supplement or prescription that will elevate this level is *real* progesterone, not progestin. In fact, you could take ten times the normal dose of progestin, and it would not raise the blood level of progesterone. When you are trying to balance or fix a deficit in progesterone, you must use progesterone.

The alarming results of a study by the Women's Health Initiative, published in the *Journal of the American Medical Association* in 2002, stirred up fear in women regarding the use of hormone replacement therapy in menopause. A portion of the study was stopped earlier than planned, due to the increased rates of breast cancer and heart disease among the group taking estrogen in combination with synthetic progesterone. The group using only estrogen continued with the study, because the same problems were not found.

Synthetic progesterone is a component of conventional HRT and was implicated in the study. Although some researchers feel that the increased cancer rates were not statistically significant, it is worth noting that the study's estrogen-only group did not show a similar increased risk of breast cancer.

When progesterone levels are testing low and a perimenopausal woman has symptoms of deficiency, I suggest that she consider using bioidentical, plant-based progesterone, which is also called "natural progesterone." The good news about natural versus synthetic progesterone/progestin is that medical professionals are starting to recognize the benefits of nonsynthetic hormones and their enhanced ability to relieve symptoms with few known side effects. Information regarding natural hormones is at an all-time high, making it easier than ever for women to have treatment alternatives.

The only prescription currently available through a non-compounding pharmacy is called *Prometrium*. Some experts contend that capsules are best,

Forms of Natural Progesterone

The natural progesterone replacement that I use in my practice requires a prescription that is formulated according to the individual dose needed. This is done at a compounding pharmacy, whose trained pharmacists understand how to formulate prescriptions into individualized regimens (see appendix A). In addition to an over-the-counter low-dose cream, natural progesterone is available in many forms:

- Capsules
- Topical creams/gels
- Drops or tablets
- Troches
- Lozenges
- Vaginal creams/gels
- Suppositories
- Rectal solutions

whereas others believe that too much progesterone is broken down when taken orally, and only a small fraction of the remainder is available for use.

I have found that sublingual drops, troches (lozenges), and topical creams are extremely effective in relieving perimenopausal symptoms in women with documented low levels of progesterone. Progesterone delivered in this way is absorbed well and effectively increases progesterone levels in the blood. Progesterone can have a sedating effect, so it is best to use it at night before going to bed. Some women prefer to take a capsule at bedtime and have good relief with the right dose. Others have found that using progesterone twice daily gives them more symptom control.

Women in their perimenopausal years can use progesterone in two ways, but the most common is to use it on a cycle.

Administering Progesterone

Days 14 through 28 of the menstrual cycle   This means that the first day of your period is always day 1 of your menstrual cycle. So fourteen days from the first day you bleed, you begin using the progesterone and continue until day 28 (or, for women with longer cycles, until your period begins). This can be adjusted to only seven or ten days before the period if necessary, and some women supplement only two or three days before the period. This is all based on severity of symptoms and is adjusted once you notice relief.

Daily, with a break for menstruation   The second most common way progesterone is administered is by using it daily with a five- to seven-day break each month. Another way to count the days would be to use it every day except those days you are having a period, or days 1 through 25 of the calendar month. This is the method most preferred by women who have had a hysterectomy but who still have their ovaries. It is also for women who are menstruating but have severe symptoms and need more coverage of progesterone.

Dosages of Natural Progesterone

Progesterone capsules   Doses range from 25 or 50 mg and from 75 to 100 mg or more. The capsules are best used at night, but they may also be used twice daily. (Typically, the dosing of capsules is higher than with creams and sublingual drops because the liver metabolizes some of the hormone.)

Progesterone drops or lozenges (sublingual)   The typical dose is 25 mg per 4 drops, or a 25, 50, 75, or 100 mg lozenge. Most patients start with 4 to 6 drops at night and 2 to 4 drops in the morning. The drops can be used on a cycle, one to two weeks prior to the period, or, if not having periods, on days 1 through 25 of the calendar month, with five to seven days off per month.

The natural progesterone drops are absorbed well under the tongue and can be flavored if necessary. Hold the drops in place with a slight wiggling of the tongue to disperse medicine for absorption. Lozenges (troches) should be held in place until they are absorbed.

Progesterone creams/gels (topical)   Rub 20 to 60 mg into the skin once or twice daily during the one to two weeks leading up to the period. The cream may also be used throughout the month, with a five- to seven-day break.

Progesterone creams are absorbed directly through the skin, just like other FDA-approved medications, such as male testosterone gels, estrogen patches, birth control patches, and pain patches. Apply the cream to thin-skinned areas, such as the inner arms, neck, face, brows, or inner thighs. I have found that most women do better on a higher-dose (3 to 10 percent) prescription cream rather than an over-the-counter preparation, which is a 1.5 to 3 percent cream. Because some women experience sleepiness when using progesterone, a smaller dose is often used in the morning.

How Do I Know If I Need Progesterone?

You may want to consider adding progesterone to your list of treatment modalities for perimenopause if any of the following apply:

▶ You have low serum (blood) or saliva progesterone levels during the second half of your menstrual cycle; or, if not menstruating, you have low levels of progesterone on two different readings through the blood or saliva.

▶ You have had a hysterectomy (whether or not ovaries have been removed) and have noticed more depression or mood swings and would like a more balanced mood with or without estrogen use.

▶ You have noted symptoms of low progesterone, with or without documented low levels of progesterone (see figure 2-4).

▶ You suffer from PMS or depression.

▶ You have symptoms of estrogen excess (see figure 2-2) or are taking estrogen and feel that you need a more balanced hormonal effect.

- ▶ You feel anxious prior to your period and have bouts of rage and anger.

- ▶ You have problems with weight gain or bloating prior to your period.

- ▶ Your periods are heavy, you have excessive cramping, or you have been diagnosed with fibroids.

- ▶ You have fibrocystic breast or chronic benign breast pain.

If you add progesterone to your treatment list, the following guidelines are recommended. Ask your medical provider to consider prescribing the dose recommended here, as many providers are not familiar with the various dosing regimes.

What to Expect When Using Progesterone

Here is what you can expect when you use progesterone for perimenopause, either during the second half of your cycle or every day except when on your period (or, if no uterus, on days 1 through 25 of the calendar month):

- ▶ Calmer, more soothing emotions, with less anger, irritability, and depression and fewer abrupt mood swings

- ▶ Fewer cravings, food binges, and blood-sugar lows

- ▶ Less cyclic weight gain

- ▶ Less bloating and water retention

- ▶ Improved sleep

- ▶ More-regular periods, with less bleeding and cramping

Keep in mind that you should work with your medical provider and report any problems or concerns that may arise as you continue with your treatment.

Troubleshooting: Progesterone

- ▶ **Little or no effect**   If you are using progesterone to help get periods back on track, or you would like lighter periods with fewer cramps, and the desired effect does not occur within two weeks of using progesterone, this may be a sign to increase your dose. I suggest raising the dose to at least one-half more during your next cycle. You will need to confer with your medical provider in this process.

- ▶ **Spotting**   If you are taking progesterone and begin spotting before your period, continue taking the progesterone until the period is due. If you start your period or have heavy bleeding while taking progesterone, stop the progesterone and count this day as day 1 of your new cycle.

▶ **No period**   If you do not get your period after taking progesterone, even at a higher dose, stop and give yourself at least two weeks off, then resume taking the progesterone. If this continues, consult your medical practitioner.

▶ **Worsening of symptoms**   When you begin taking progesterone, it is possible that your symptoms may become worse for the first two weeks. This is an occasional response and seems to happen with women who also have long-standing progesterone deficiency and estrogen dominance. Please stick with it, or lower your dose and then gradually increase it over the next several cycles.

Estrogen Therapy in Perimenopause

Most women consider estrogen a prescription reserved strictly for menopause, even though commonly prescribed birth control pills contain higher levels of estrogen than what is discussed here. As noted earlier, perimenopause means "around menopause." It is safe to say that around menopause many women intermittently or cyclically have low levels of estrogen. This can be a rocky time for many women whose estrogen levels are all over the chart. Estrogen can help relieve symptoms that are not relieved by progesterone alone. A week after ovulation, estrogen and progesterone levels fall; and in perimenopause this drop can be abrupt and cause unpleasant symptoms. Medical providers often prescribe birth control pills as a leveler; and while this can work for some, it may cause unwanted side effects in others.

It is important that estrogen levels are evaluated appropriately during the second half of the cycle. If a woman does not have periods due to a hysterectomy, conducting two different tests two weeks apart can be helpful in pinpointing the exact hormonal ebb and flow. In addition, the symptoms should be of estrogen deficiency, not estrogen excess, to treat with estrogen.

When Is Estrogen Helpful?

Estrogen is useful for three situations during perimenopause when there are documented levels of estrogen deficiency.

▶ Intermittent fluctuations of symptoms. This could include hot flashes two days before the onset of the period. It could also include symptoms such as insomnia that may occur throughout the week before the period.

▶ Symptoms throughout the entire cycle. Women lose approximately 30 percent of their estrogen by the time they hit perimenopause. Most women adapt well with diet and lifestyle alternations, stress reduction, and, in some cases, by using progesterone. It has been my experience, however, that some women need to add estrogen to the plan to finally get control of their symptoms.

▶ Temporary symptoms of estrogen deficiency. This includes women who have never had symptoms of estrogen deficiency, but all of a sudden find themselves symptomatic with low estrogen levels in the second half of the cycle. These women may need only two or three months of treatment to boost their estrogen production and then are able to stop the treatment. I have found that these women have a significant improvement if they also seek other areas of treatment through diet, exercise, and stress management.

The goal with estrogen is to help the woman become symptom-free throughout the cycle and to increase estrogen levels into the normal range. Again, what may be normal for one woman may not be normal for another, so elevating a woman's estrogen into the high-normal range may be perfect for some, whereas others may need to be nudged only into the middle or low ranges.

Again, natural estrogen replacement therapies are preferred because of their bioidentical properties and also because fine-tuning can be done at a compounding pharmacy with doses adjusted as necessary throughout the treatment period. Following are suggestions for estrogen treatment cyclically in perimenopause.

Estrogen can be used in the following fashions for perimenopause:

▶ From ovulation until the onset of period, two weeks prior to the period.

▶ Two days to one week prior to the period.

▶ At a low dose throughout the month. This is particularly helpful for women who have had a hysterectomy and have ongoing symptoms of estrogen deficiency, but have levels that are borderline low. It is also important to remember that most medical providers suggest a low-dose birth control pill for perimenopausal symptoms, which contain far more estrogen than the natural alternatives. It is important to monitor estrogen levels when being treated with estrogen.

▶ Estrogen should be accompanied with progesterone to protect the uterus from excessive buildup in the lining and potentially increasing the risk for abnormal uterine cells. Progesterone also increases the effectiveness of estrogen by stimulating estrogen receptors.

Natural Estrogen Choices

Here are some suggestions for supplementing estrogen during perimenopause.

Tri-Estrogen   A *tri-estrogen* incorporates all three types of estrogen—estriol, estradiol, and estrone—but has the greatest amount of estriol. Estriol is the least potent of the three and has been found in some smaller studies to be breast protective. Tri-estrogen is plant-based and is available only by prescription from a compounding pharmacy. The breakdown is typically 80 percent estriol, 10 percent estrone, and 10 percent estradiol, but other combinations are available, and the three estrogens can be combined in numerous ways.

Estradiol is the most potent of the estrogens. My experience is that it has the greatest effect on symptom relief for hot flashes, insomnia, headaches, mental fogginess, and fatigue.

Although *estrone* is the most prevalent estrogen in menopause, I choose not to replace with this estrogen. There is some concern that estrone metabolizes into a harmful and potential cancer-causing estrogen and, in my opinion, is not necessary in the mix.

Estriol, being the weakest and most likely the safest estrogen, can cause a woman to feel bloated or to gain fat around the middle, but it may be the estrogen of choice for women at high risk for breast cancer. Despite these possible effects, I prescribe this estrogen because it is effective in protecting the vagina from dryness and the bladder from incontinence-related problems.

If the combination is correct and is not predominantly estriol, most of my patients do not experience abdominal bloating. The compounding pharmacist can be of great assistance in determining the appropriate combination for you and can work cooperatively with your medical provider.

Bi-Estrogen   A *bi-estrogen* incorporates two types of estrogen—estriol and estradiol. The breakdown with bi-estrogen could be 30 to 60 percent estradiol and 30 to 60 percent estriol.

A bi-estrogen may be prescribed if bloating occurs with tri-estrogen or if greater relief of premenopausal symptoms is needed. The breakdown of bi-estrogen could be 60 percent estradiol and 40 percent estriol, which would give you the greatest effect on symptom relief, but is a more potent estrogen prescription. Another option could be 70 percent estriol and 30 percent estradiol, which is still excellent for symptom relief but is milder in its estrogen effect.

Dosages of Natural Estrogen

Tri-estrogen or bi-estrogen capsules   Doses range from 0.75 to 1.75 mg per capsule. Start with one capsule daily and increase to twice daily if necessary, one in the morning and one at bedtime.

Tri-estrogen or bi-estrogen drops (sublingual)   The typical dose is 0.625 mg per drop. Start with 1 to 2 drops twice daily. This will help with mild symptoms such as occasional hot flashes, headaches, mental confusion, reduced memory, and insomnia. If symptoms are more severe, 2 to 4 drops twice daily may be needed. Place drops under the tongue daily or just during the one to two weeks before the period.

Tri-estrogen or bi-estrogen creams/gels (topical)   The typical strength is 1 mg per gram of gel or cream. Rub 0.5 g of gel or cream into the skin twice daily. (The compounding pharmacist will give directions on what the volume is in each specific prescription.) The amount can vary, but typically women should start with only one application daily and increase from there only if necessary. See chapter 10 for using estrogen combinations with specific hormonal problems, such as headaches, hot flashes, PMS, or estrogen deficiency before the period.

Synthetic Estrogen Alternatives

Estrogen patch   This prescription is filled at a traditional pharmacy rather than a compounding pharmacy. The patch is often a good option, as the dose can be very low and absorption through the skin is often preferred for women with mild symptoms. The patch can be used once or twice weekly, as it delivers a continuous low dose of estrogen throughout the week. Starting with a 0.25 mg dose and increasing to a 0.375 or 0.50 mg dose if necessary during the two weeks before the period is often all that is needed to relieve persistent perimenopausal symptoms. The patch can be used just before the period to help with falling levels of estrogen or when progesterone alone has not been effective.

Birth control pills   The pill can help with fluctuating perimenopausal symptoms and make a difference in a woman's day-to-day balance; but for some women who do not tolerate chemical substitutes (or synthetic progesterone in the pill), this is not a good option. The pill may add protection against uterine and ovarian cancer. It also preserves fertility and reduces some gynecological hazards, such as heavy, cramping periods and endometriosis. The downside to using the pill is that it reduces circulating levels of testosterone, causing some women to have symptoms of testosterone deficiency, including low libido.

Additional Alternatives for Correcting Estrogen Balance

If after reading the symptom list in figure 2-2 you suspect that you have high estrogen levels, or estrogen dominance, I suggest the following treatment guidelines. If you have signs of low estrogen, and testing supports it, this section offers additional comments about getting balanced. Note that by first treating other low-level hormones, such as testosterone or progesterone, you

How to Use Estrogen While Still Having Periods

- Use estrogen the week before the period and into the first four to five days of the period, if necessary, to relieve symptoms.

- Do not use estrogen during the second week of the cycle unless you have been diagnosed with low levels of estrogen throughout the cycle. During the second week of the cycle (around ovulation), you are typically producing the most estrogen.

- After using estrogen replacement for a while, it is possible that you may start producing adequate amounts of estrogen on your own. You may also start producing adequate estrogen after improving your diet, reducing stress, and getting regular exercise. If this is the case, estrogen replacement could be stopped.

- The symptoms of too much estrogen include sore breasts, bloating, water retention, increased breast size, irritability, cramping, and nausea. (See figure 2-2 for a complete list.)

If you notice these symptoms, reduce your intake to one-half dose for two weeks. If symptoms continue, schedule a blood test to evaluate your hormone levels. After using estrogen for a while, it is possible that you will no longer need it, especially if you have made positive lifestyle changes that enhance natural hormone production.

may actually correct estrogen levels without needing to resort to estrogen use. A 60-day follow-up test to see if estrogen is really needed would be in order.

Bioidentical progesterone   The use of bioidentical progesterone is extremely helpful in creating a more normal balance. *Bioidentical* means that it is identical in molecular structure to the human body's progesterone. Although it is plant-based, bioidentical progesterone is far more valuable in treating symptoms because the body recognizes the progesterone as its own type. It can be taken as a capsule, a sublingual lozenge, or drops, or as a cream/gel that is absorbed through the skin.

High-fiber diet   A diet high in fiber is healthy for numerous reasons and will help bind excessive estrogen for elimination. Several studies have documented that fiber can bind up to 30 percent of the excess estrogen in the intestinal tract.

Calcium d-glucarate   A twice-daily supplement of 400 mg of calcium d-glucarate can help by blocking the beta-glucuronidase activity in the gut. This activity is responsible for allowing your system to reactivate estrogen and move it back into the bloodstream. This recycling process of moving estrogen into the bloodstream instead of sending it out as waste is how the body retains unnecessary estrogen.

Weight loss   Lose weight or reduce body fat. Fat cells, especially those around the midsection, produce enzymes that increase estrogen levels in the blood.

Phytoestrogens   Take 100 to 250 mg per day of isoflavones, which compete with the estrogen receptors, thus reducing blood estrogen levels. Though it may not be necessary to overindulge in phytoestrogens, specialists in women's healthcare commonly believe that phytoestrogens improve estrogen metabolism by blocking estrogen sites.

Zinc   Taking 30 to 50 mg per day of this natural aromatase inhibitor (estrogen receptor blocker) will help to reduce excessive estrogen production.

Reducing alcohol intake   Reducing or eliminating alcohol consumption will improve liver function, enabling it to efficiently eliminate excess estrogen.

Getting your liver in shape   Most women do not understand the importance of the liver with respect to hormonal balance. One of the liver's responsibilities is to deactivate and excrete estrogen at the end of the estrogen cycle. Keeping the liver functioning well allows for healthier metabolism and elimination of excess estrogen. Review your current medications that may interfere with healthy liver function. Common drugs that interfere with estrogen metabolism and elimination include ibuprofen, anti-inflammatories, aspirin, cholesterol-lowering drugs, some heart and blood-pressure drugs, esophageal reflux medications, and some antidepressants.

Here are some additional supplements to improve liver function:

▶ Take inositol and choline (100 mg each daily).

▶ Take the amino acids methionine (150 mg) and n-acetyl cysteine (250 to 500 mg) daily.

▶ Take the antioxidant alpha lipoic acid (500 mg twice daily).

▶ Take the supplement known as DIM, or indole-3-carbinol (400 to 800 mg daily), which is extremely beneficial in protecting against estrogen dominance by improving the elimination of excessive estrogen.

Liver Flush Cocktail

Your liver is a workhorse that works overtime most of the day. When it lacks the correct nutrients and is overcome by toxins from the environment, food, stress, or other factors, it no longer works with great enthusiasm. At that point your skin becomes ruddy, and you may notice more cellulite, abdominal bloating, indigestion, high blood pressure, fatigue, mood swings, and depression. When your liver is sluggish, every organ in your body can be affected. Whenever this happens, consider a cocktail to help flush out toxins and support the functioning of your liver. Here is a basic recipe:

In a blender combine:

8 oz. distilled or purified water or seasonal fresh fruit juice
1 clove garlic
1 tablespoon cold-pressed olive oil
1-inch piece of fresh ginger root

Blend well and drink straight (don't sip).

▶ Take a liver detox supplement such as milk thistle or a combination supplement found in health food stores.

▶ Take garlic and ginger root, either in cooking or in the form of a "cocktail" (see "Liver Flush Cocktail").

▶ Taking 1 to 2 tablespoons of flaxseed oil per day can also help. Studies have shown that deficiencies of omega-3 fatty acids can create menopausal symptoms and hormone fluctuations.

What About Testosterone?

Gone are the days of thinking that testosterone is just a "guy thing." Female ovaries produce testosterone, which decreases dramatically from original levels by a woman's thirties and forties. As discussed in detail in chapter 2, testosterone helps with the following:

▶ Sex drive and sensation

▶ Endurance and muscle strength

▶ Leaner body, with less fat

▶ Improved balance and coordination

▶ Increased energy

Doesn't sound half-bad, does it? When a woman shows signs of testosterone deficiency, and blood levels return very low, it is possible that she needs to supplement with low, female-sized doses of testosterone. I emphasize the *female* part because it is important for women to know that the goal is still to avoid the possible acne, excess hairiness, and lower voice associated with larger, male-sized doses.

Testosterone is a prescription hormone that is being researched heavily for use by women. Today there is just one testosterone-only prescription that works well for women with few side effects: natural testosterone. It can be used as a cream, as sublingual drops, as a lozenge, or as a capsule. It can also be combined with other hormones to reduce the cost and improve the compliance of taking it. Once you are stabilized on a dose, you will not need to change doses frequently.

Typically, by age fifty women have lost approximately 50 percent of the testosterone production that they had at age twenty. The amount that each woman loses is variable and depends on such factors as lifestyle, strength training, current muscle mass, body fat, and genetics.

Women who naturally have high estrogen levels, or who are taking too much estrogen, may have very low levels of testosterone. Estrogen increases a protein called *sex hormone–binding globulin (SHBG),* which binds up testosterone. When you use testosterone and progesterone to reduce estrogen dominance, there will come a time when you will need to either reduce the testosterone or stop it altogether; once your body comes into natural balance, more ovarian testosterone is being made, even as less sex hormone–binding globulin is being produced. The take-home message is that you need to watch your levels carefully by testing every three to six months.

Things to Remember When Using Testosterone Replacement

■ You should monitor how you feel with the testosterone. Its benefits can be subtle, so it is important to be honest when evaluating your response. Notice your levels of energy and sexual desire. Most likely you will not experience a sudden surge; you more likely will gradually feel more interested rather than repulsed at the prospect of having sex. Other things to take into consideration are your mood, endurance, muscle tone, strength and coordination, and memory.

■ If you have symptoms of excess testosterone—acne, facial hair growth, irritability, weight gain, and aggressiveness—I recommend reducing your dose by half or using it only every other day. This will help bring your level down, and you can gradually increase the dose if necessary. Some women need very little testosterone to increase their blood levels, whereas others are resistant. Be mindful of the potential side effects of testosterone excess. Although it is uncommon to see these symptoms with the low doses that are used, watch for them nonetheless. Blood tests for testosterone levels should be ordered every three to six months.

■ If you have high testosterone levels when initially evaluated and have had long-term problems with testosterone excess, I suggest trying *Aldactone,* a common medication used to reduce testosterone levels. It is often used in the treatment of polycystic ovarian syndrome and is known as an "anti-androgen." This medication can reduce circulating levels of testosterone and therefore relieve symptoms of excess.

Dosages of Testosterone

Testosterone capsules   The capsules are available in variable strengths. Start with 2 to 4 mg once or twice daily. Most women take the capsule only in the morning, and the dosage can be increased as necessary.

Testosterone drops (sublingual)   These drops are available in many doses. The potency of the testosterone is 1 mg per drop. I recommend starting on 1 to 2 drops twice daily and, if necessary, using it thirty minutes before intercourse. Exceeding 10 drops per day is not recommended unless the patient has been evaluated and repeat blood levels are drawn.

Testosterone creams/gels (topical)   Rub 1 to 3 mg into the skin once daily. I recommend applying to the upper inner thighs, the inner labia (genital area), or in the pubic area. Rubbing the cream into the genital area serves two purposes. First, it will help distribute the cream into the pelvic area, which can strengthen the bladder muscles and sex organs. The second reason is that a small percentage of women will have some local hair growth where they apply the cream, so using it in the genital area makes sense. In addition, applying the testosterone to the clitoral area five to ten minutes prior to intercourse can increase the strength of orgasm and improve sexual sensation for some women. If using it in the genital area, to avoid irritation ask for a gel or cream that can be applied to the genital area.

Moving Forward with Hormonal Balance

It is important that each woman understand that balancing hormones is a *process* and that she is a unique individual who requires a treatment plan based on her own profile and symptoms. Adjustments are almost always necessary during the course of treatment, and patience and mindfulness to your responses are essential for achieving optimal hormonal balance. Do not be discouraged if you experience side effects to the hormones or if you have not felt completely in control of your symptoms after the first attempt at treatment. Adjustments in even the smallest doses can make a dramatic difference in how you feel.

Chapter 5

Fix Your Diet: The Most Powerful Way to Create Hormonal Balance

IN THIS CHAPTER:

Why Women Gain Weight with Age

A Six-Step Plan for Weight/Fat Loss

Tips for Success

Exercise Your Way to a Lean Body

Forty-four-year-old Angie thought she must have been gaining weight by the second. She came to my office distraught and confessed that she felt that her food cravings and eating habits were out of control. Angie had tried various diet plans and would lose five or ten pounds only to gain them back. She continually put off buying new clothes because she wasn't at her desired weight, but after several years her clothes were becoming threadbare!

Angie had a stressful job and, as the single mom of two active children, had precious little time to spare. What with getting the kids up and ready each morning, it's no wonder that she rarely ate breakfast. She had skipped it so often that she had convinced herself that the habit was beneficial—no breakfast, no calories. Midday she would grab a little something for lunch, even though she was hungry enough to eat a full meal. Again, she was giving herself license to overeat later. By 6 p.m. the woman was an eating machine.

Even though she didn't say "The devil made me do it," Angie was at a loss as to what *was* making her Hoover through her refrigerator and cupboards every night. She would eat a full meal while fixing dinner, then eat another meal when dinner was on the table. Later she'd rummage around the kitchen, looking for a little something to top off the night, just a little snack—like two bowls of ice cream. She was so busy at night trying to get things done for the next day that she was hardly aware of her almost constant munching.

In evaluating her habits, I showed Angie that she was consuming 85 percent of her calories after 6 p.m. She was hungry, but she was also eating to calm herself after a hard day and soothe her nerves for the next round. She'd developed this pattern over the years and didn't question it. Angie loved food and felt emotionally tied to the boost that it provided.

Angie was a hard case, but she is now in control of her life—and her eating. Her four daily meals kick off with a quick protein breakfast shake with fruit and are interspersed with at least eight glasses of water every day. She exercises first thing in the morning, alternating her treadmill with flexible-band strength training and a Pilates workout. She is thrilled that she has more energy now than fifteen years ago and that she fits into jeans she wore in her twenties. All told, it takes Angie about forty minutes each day to prepare her food and exercise. She figures that forty minutes is a small price to pay for feeling and looking so much better. If Angie can find forty minutes to put the information in this chapter to work, so can you! Maybe it's time…

Why Women Gain Weight with Age

Does it seem as though you're eating about the same as when you were younger, but you keep piling on the pounds, especially around the middle? Or maybe you've never had a weight problem, but since you hit forty fat is bulging or jiggling in places you never dreamed that it would. I have experienced this frustration firsthand. If I had to name one thing that upsets women in their forties the most, it is this inexplicable weight gain. If increasing girth and the maddening development of an abdominal spare tire bewilders you, read this chapter—it can set you on the path to change your life!

There is one primary force at work here: *insulin resistance;* that's when insulin, usually your good buddy, becomes your personal fat-storage hormone. Researcher and scientist Barry Sears, Ph.D., has shown how we store fat and produce excess insulin in direct response to our diet. In his book *Enter the Zone,* Dr. Sears explains the body's specific chemical reactions to food. The process is simple: If your diet is sparse on protein and heavy on refined carbohydrates, such as breads, pasta, bagels, crackers, desserts, candy, sweet snacks, and non-diet soft drinks, you are most likely storing fat at an accelerated rate right around the middle. And it matters little if desserts and snacks are so-called low fat.

A high-carbohydrate diet also induces exhaustion, especially in the late afternoon; increased food cravings, usually at around 4 p.m. and after dinner; irritability and low moods or depression; and bloating and water retention. Sound familiar? The process goes something like this: When we eat, the glucose from our food is transported to the cells for storage. Insulin, produced by the pancreas, is the key hormone to open the cell doors for glucose storage. Unfortunately, individuals who overload on foods that raise insulin levels overproduce the hormone, causing "resistance" at the cellular level.

This is a problem because when the cells in the muscles, nervous system, and organs close their doors to the high levels of insulin in the blood, the body compensates by stashing the glucose in other areas, resulting in increased fat storage. Over time even the fat cells become resistant, and the blood sugar has nowhere to go. When excess blood sugar remains in the bloodstream, the diabetes epidemic in the United States claims another victim.

We live in a society that adores bready foods—and in great quantities. You know, those steaming mountains of linguine and spaghetti, softball-sized muffins and bagels, double-sized donuts, and Twinkies two to the pack. We love our baskets of breadsticks, garlic bread by the yard, and double-crust pizza. For snacks we'll stuff down a bag of chips or a plate-sized piece of cake. All these foods are basically sugar and flour, which begin converting to glucose the minute they enter our mouths. Too much glucose puts the pancreas into overdrive, overproducing insulin to help control rising blood-sugar levels. The pancreas is in a frenzy of fruitless production, and if glucose overload continues, it will simply refuse to work. Then you've got diabetes.

The signs of insulin resistance are the same as those for low blood-sugar (hypoglycemia); they include irritability, shakiness, fatigue, intense cravings, confusion, headaches, and increased fat around the middle.

In short when the diet is too heavy in refined, starch-laden carbohydrates at the expense of too little protein, vegetables, and fruits, sugar levels rise, excess insulin is produced, and we move quickly to a fat-storage zone. We don't want to go there. Sadly, our bodies become more naturally insulin resistant as we age, predisposing us to weight gain and partially explaining irksome peri-menopausal abdominal fat storage.

What's more, as our ovaries naturally produce less estrogen during perimenopause, the body's fat cells gear up to produce more. Didn't realize that fat cells produce estrogen? They do. That's the primary reason why being overweight is a risk factor for estrogen-sensitive cancers, such as certain breast cancers.

The perimenopausal body strives for hormonal balance, even going so far as to multiply the number of fat cells and to increase their size, especially around the waistline. In her book *Take Charge of the Change,* author Pamela Smith, R.D., says that the fat cells often begin to accumulate in the perimenopausal years due to estrogen fluctuations; but once hormonal balance is restored, the fat-storage zone can be replaced with a fat-*burning* zone. Smith adds that the midlife fat cell production need not be inevitable for women, nor is it impossible to control. Forgoing strict dieting and deprivation and beginning to live in a new and balanced way will unlock the fat cell doors so shrinking can once again take place. Then there's the unpleasant fact that women lose muscle mass during middle age at the same time they're gaining fat. Muscles burn calories, and the greater the muscle mass, the more revved up the body's metabolism. Fat, on the other hand, just hangs there and does nothing to boost metabolism. Don't despair, however; the situation is far from hopeless.

A Six-Step Plan for Weight/Fat Loss

The plan outlined below will help reduce fat, improve energy, elevate mood, slow aging, and reverse insulin resistance.

Do not try to make the dietary and lifestyle changes any harder—just remember how our ancestors ate. Most likely they didn't have a donut and coffee for breakfast, a bagel at midmorning, and a burger and fries for lunch. Of course, unlike us, they weren't plagued by diabetes, obesity, depression, and hormonal imbalances.

After you consult your medical provider about the need to lose body fat, I suggest that the following steps be gradually incorporated.

Step 1: Eat Protein

It is time to let protein be your friend. Gone are the days of thinking that protein is bad because it is "high fat." Lean proteins are brain food and muscle fuel. Without protein we lose muscle mass, reduce metabolism, and gain weight. With insufficient protein we can feel restless, tired, and emotional. Add protein to each meal in the form of eggs, fish, low-fat turkey, chicken, pork, lamb, or lean beef. Dairy products contain protein, but stick to low-fat products. Soy products such as tofu are excellent sources of protein, as are certain grain and

High-Protein, Low-Fat Snacks

- Hard-boiled egg (75 cal., 5 g fat, 6 g protein)
- Water-packed tuna, lightly salted (3.5 oz.: 131 cal., 1 g fat, 30 g protein) on celery and/or whole-grain crackers
- Baked potato with Yogurt Cream Cheese (on page 68)
- Cooked shrimp (3.5 oz.: 99 cal., 1 g fat, 21 g protein)
- Skim milk (½ cup: 70 cal., 1 g fat, 3 g protein)
- Cottage cheese 1 percent (½ cup: 72 cal., 1 g fat, 12 g protein)
- Plain fat-free yogurt (½ cup: 63 cal., 2 g fat, 5 g protein)
- Almonds (1 oz.: 168 cal., 14 g fat, 8 g protein)
- Dry-roasted peanuts (1 oz.: 162 cal., 14 g fat, 7.5 g protein)

legume combinations that form complete proteins. (See "High-Protein, Low-Fat Snacks" and "High-Protein, Healthy Snacks."

Step 2: Eliminate Sugar

Pure and simple: Just get it out of your diet if you want to lose body fat. By *sugar* I mean candy and sweets, of course, but also starchy processed foods that begin their conversion to glucose the instant they pass your lips. If you are trying to reduce fat and fatigue, have no more than two starchy carbohydrates per day, and keep them as unrefined as possible. Baked potatoes with the skin or a slice of sprouted wheat bread are good choices—not bagels, chips, crackers, and heaping bowls of pasta. (See "High-Protein, Low-Fat Snacks.")

High-Protein, Healthy Snacks

- Nachos: 0.5 oz. baked tortilla chips, 1 tablespoon salsa, 1 oz. low-fat jack cheese, 1 tablespoon avocado
- Ham, fruit, and nuts: 4 slices 97 percent fat-free ham, half an apple or other fruit, 8 to 10 macadamia nuts
- Low-fat cottage cheese, fruit, and nuts: ¼ cup low-fat cottage cheese, canned light fruit, 8 to 10 almonds
- Cheese, grapes, and nuts: 1 oz. part skim mozzarella string cheese, ½ cup grapes, handful of peanuts

Step 3: Eat Your Fruits and Veggies

Aim for five servings of vegetables per day, and eat two fruits per day. Fresh is best and juice doesn't count. Here's a rule of thumb: The more highly colored a fruit or vegetable, the better it is for you. Iceberg lettuce hardly counts as a vegetable. Deeply green kale, chard, and spinach, on the other hand, are loaded with vitamins and minerals. (See "Many Veggie Soup," "Salad Tips," and "Salad Dressing: The Silent Saboteur.")

Many-Veggie Soup

This simple recipe for no-fat, high-vitamin soup is a lifesaver. It's delicious, fills you up, and gives you your daily five in one bowl! It's great for lunch and for taking the edge off before the evening, so you don't fill up on starches.

- 6 cups broth, vegetable or low-sodium, nonfat chicken or beef
- 2 cups chopped green cabbage
- 2 carrots, peeled, cut into ½-inch pieces
- 2 stalks celery, cut into ½-inch pieces
- 1 small onion, diced
- 1 clove garlic, minced
- 1 cup cut green beans
- 1 16-ounce can diced tomatoes, or 3 Roma tomatoes, peeled and chopped
- 1 teaspoon each dried thyme, basil, and oregano
- 2 small zucchini, split lengthwise and cut into ½-inch slices
- ¼ cup chopped parsley
- 1 cup packed fresh small spinach leaves
- Salt and pepper to taste
- Optional (see *Note* below): 1 medium red or white rose potato, peeled, diced; or 1 cup corn kernels; or 1 cup cooked dried beans

Place the broth in a large soup pot. Add the cabbage, carrots, celery, onion, garlic, and green beans. Drain the tomato juices into the mixture. Add the dried herbs, and bring the pot to a boil. Turn the heat down once the pot is bubbling, and allow to simmer for about 15 minutes. Add the zucchini and parsley, and cook another 10 minutes. Drop in the spinach leaves, season with salt and pepper, and taste to adjust the seasonings.

Note: If you choose to add the potatoes, corn, or cooked beans, add them with the zucchini and parsley. This nutritious, delicious, forgiving soup can accept almost any vegetable you have on hand, but add strongly flavored ones only sparingly. Vegetables like broccoli, cauliflower, and turnips can too easily dominate the lively flavors of the other vegetables.

Salad Tips

- Always order salad dressing on the side.
- Dip the tip of the fork in the dressing, then spear a bite of salad.
- Use low-fat alternatives such as rice wine vinegar, lemon juice, or commercially blended balsamic vinegars.

Salad Dressing: The Silent Saboteur

Nothing sabotages a diet more surreptitiously than salad dressing. You opt for the green salad in lieu of the cheeseburger—a savings of about 1,000 calories and 40 grams of fat—but then negate your good deed by dumping 500 calories worth of condiments on it!

There are many delicious alternatives to fat- and sugar-laden bottled salad dressings, such as the following, simple homemade versions.

Vinaigrettes   Place the following ingredients in a screw-top jar and shake to blend well. You'll have on hand a simple and very low fat salad dressing that will be deliciously satisfying to sprinkle on your salads with guilt-free abandon.

Raspberry Vinaigrette

- 2 tablespoons of nonfat yogurt or fat-free sour cream
- ¼ cup of raspberry vinegar
- 1 teaspoon minced chives
- 1 teaspoon fresh mint leaves

If you have them, add a few spoonfuls of crushed fresh raspberries, otherwise consider adding a ½ teaspoon of poppy seeds. This is especially nice with a fresh fruit salad.

Herbed Vinaigrette

- ¼ cup red wine vinegar
- ¼ cup tomato or mixed vegetable juice
- 1 tablespoon water
- 1 tablespoon olive oil
- ½ teaspoon each of oregano, thyme, and chives
- 1 crushed clove of garlic
- ½ teaspoon black pepper

Citrus Vinaigrette I

- Juice of 1 fresh orange (about 4 ounces)
- 4 tablespoons fresh grapefruit juice
- 2 tablespoons fresh lemon or lime juice
- 1 tablespoon olive oil
- 1 tablespoon honey
- 1 tablespoon Dijon mustard
- 1 tablespoon low-sodium soy sauce
- 2 teaspoons crushed fresh ginger root (use a garlic press)

Citrus Vinaigrette II

- ¾ cup orange juice
- ¼ cup lime juice
- ¼ cup finely chopped fresh basil leaves
- 1 tablespoon olive oil
- 1 teaspoon Dijon mustard
- Dash salt

Step 4: Drink Water

Drink eight to ten 8-ounce glasses of water per day. To simplify, fill a clean half-gallon milk jug with water and make it a goal to drink it all. Adding lemon or sugar-free flavorings may make it more interesting. Water speeds up your metabolism, wakes you up during the day, relieves tired muscles, prevents injuries, reduces wrinkles, and works to eliminate headaches. Do you need any more reason to get enough water?

Step 5: Incorporate "Good Fat"

Include small amounts of good fat to your diet. Try adding a handful of walnuts, almonds, sunflower seeds, or olives every day. Walnuts are best because they raise your good cholesterol. When preparing recipes, use olive, canola, or flaxseed oil. You need good fat for a healthy heart and, ironically, to *lose* fat. You don't need much, but you do need at least one to two tablespoons every day. Fat also increases satisfaction with food, tiding us over until it's time to eat again. It also improves our skin and reduces hair loss.

Yogurt Cream Cheese

This excellent, fat-free faux cream cheese may be seasoned with a wide variety of herbs or other additions. Spread on whole-grain crackers or stuff into celery; it's really good! Add it with steamed broccoli flowerets to a baked potato and skip the butter and sour cream. A softer version of the cheese is much like sour cream and makes a lovely, guilt-free dip for raw veggies.

Place 8 ounces of fat-free yogurt into a fine cloth strainer (or you may improvise using a small plastic coffee cone and a paper coffee filter, which works equally well). Place the strainer over a bowl to catch the liquid that drains off. Cover with plastic wrap and place in the refrigerator. Let it sit at least 4 hours or overnight. The length of time the yogurt drains will determine the consistency of the finished cheese—the longer it sits, the firmer the cheese will be.

When it reaches the desired consistency, unmold it onto a plate or into a bowl and season it as you wish. Try adding chopped fresh herbs, alone or in combination: basil, thyme, tarragon, mint, oregano, and chives. Crushed garlic and minced sun-dried tomatoes make a delicious version. A sweeter variation is very good on a fresh fruit salad. You can also blend the thickened yogurt with crushed fresh berries or other chopped soft fruit such as peaches, apricots, or nectarines.

Step 6: Get Moving!

Exercise is essential for long-term weight loss and for a healthy, longer life. If you are depressed about how you feel, start exercising daily and you will feel amazingly better about yourself within days! (See "Simple Exercises for Improved Body Image" in chapter 8.)

Tips for Success

Don't try to overhaul your lifestyle overnight   Instead, take small, incremental steps. If you master just one change per month, in six months you'll have it all put together. Perhaps start by adding protein to your breakfast and committing to a 20-minute walk every evening with your partner or a friend.

Keep a detailed food diary   Try documenting your food intake for five to seven days. If you feel you are already doing everything right and are still not seeing results, this can be quite revealing. If you constantly sample food while cooking or clean up leftovers from the kids' plates, for example, you could be consuming hundreds of extra calories. Studies show that the average person actually consumes in excess of 500 calories more than he or she estimates.

Mix up your aerobic activity   Try something new every two to three weeks, and gradually increase the time spent exercising—up to 45 minutes per session. If you haven't added weight-resistance training, now is the time! You could also substitute one of your aerobic/cardio workouts for a strength-training workout. Muscle burns fat! (See "Simple Exercises for Improved Body Image" in chapter 8.)

Remember the protein   Eating high-protein foods will help you stay satisfied so you're not tempted to gorge on junk. Include some protein with each meal.

Be happy with losing 1 to 2 pounds per week   If you do this for two months, you will be down up to 16 pounds. Gradual weight loss will keep the pounds off better than crash diets. That's when it counts, so stick with it!

Take one free day per week   That's right—one free day! You deserve a day that is set aside for what you really want to eat or drink. The catch here is *six days on and one day off.* Try to make at least 75 percent of your week on track; that way, if you go off your plan or have a slip-up, you can get right back into it so that no more than 25 percent of your week is off. A great plan is to have Sunday through Friday be your good days, and Saturday your "reward day." You may be thinking, *This sounds a little too easy—and like too much food for weight loss.* All I can say is try it and you'll see. Your body will like it and so will you!

Simple Steps to Support Your Efforts

Read labels   Keep sugar grams low (fewer than 5 to 10 g per serving). Beware of extremely high carbohydrate content, trans-fatty acids, and saturated fats. Combined with sugar, fats are a sure-fire way of sending your insulin level up and causing fat storage supreme!

Eat regularly   Your engine needs fuel to keep running. Ever wonder why some people can't lose weight by skipping meals or restricting food intake? Even if you eat practically nothing throughout the day and then eat a sensible dinner, you will have a more difficult time losing fat and keeping it off than if you ate small amounts over the course of the day. When you feel hungry, your metabolism switches to slow burn to conserve energy. Keep your engine stoked by eating four or five times a day.

Many types of protein bars or shakes are convenient and nutritious. Snacking with protein at 3 or 4 p.m. can help to control nighttime noshing. A recent study compared two groups of people on a calorie-restricted plan. One group consumed the calories in two meals per day, and the other group ate them over five meals. After twelve weeks the group that ate two meals per day lost weight—but it was muscle weight. The group that ate five meals per day also lost weight—but it was *all fat!* This is a perfect example of how important it is to eat throughout the day. You need your muscle for metabolism, and losing the fat will transform your body quickly!

Eat breakfast   Studies show that eating breakfast can increase your metabolism and help you burn up to 10 percent more calories throughout the day. Start your morning with protein and a non-sugary carbohydrate such as fruit or oatmeal.

Stifle the evening snacking   Have you been eating ice cream or popcorn before bed and then wake up feeling tired or headachy? Surprise! It's your insulin level up all night, just for you! Pre-sleep snacking may work for hibernating bears, but it's no way to keep from storing fat during the night.

Clean out your refrigerator and cupboards   If it's there, you will most likely find it and eat it. Don't tempt yourself! Get rid of the snack foods that will call your name. We wouldn't think of putting alcohol in front of a recovering alcoholic, so why keep foods that are addicting in your own kitchen? Your family doesn't need them either.

Commit to this plan and stick with it   Try to refocus on your goals daily by visualizing what it is you desire. Picture your fit, energetic self, and remember to recommit daily to your new lifestyle to keep it a priority. Pray for the power to stick with it.

Quit the negative self-talk   We were not designed to constantly tell ourselves how ugly, fat, useless, out-of-control, big-butted, and gigantic-thighed we are without eventually believing it! In time it becomes a self-fulfilling prophecy. So why not tell yourself you are beautiful, alive, in control, moving forward, shaping up, wonderfully made, and becoming healthier. Say it enough times, believe it, and it will be true!

Supplements for Weight/Fat Loss

Supplements can help balance your blood sugar and reduce your cravings, while at the same time increasing your energy.

Chromium picolinate (200–800 mcg per day)   Chromium picolinate helps balance unstable blood-sugar levels and possibly reduce cravings. It is excellent for women who are sugar sensitive or diabetic.

Flaxseed oil capsules (2,000–6,000 mg per day with food)
Flaxseed oil provides omega-3 fatty acids that help with fat metabolism, appetite, and healthiness of skin, hair, and nails, while helping protect the heart.

L-carnitine (500–2,000 mg per day)   L-carnitine helps metabolize fat and reduce cravings.

Siberian ginseng (500 mg, 2 or 3 times per day)   Ginseng provides a feeling of fullness. It also gives energy and helps curb the appetite.

Co-enzyme Q_{10} (50–250 mg per day)   Co-enzyme Q_{10} helps boost metabolism and has been shown to reduce heart disease.

L-glutamine (500–1,000 mg per day)   This supplement may help with cravings and blood-sugar balance. I have found it helpful in curbing sugar cravings.

Exercise Your Way to a Lean Body

I would not be doing this chapter justice if I let you off without enlightening you on the unbelievably positive benefits of exercise, which every perimeno-pausal woman needs. It's beneficial not only for burning fat, but also for your emotions, stress relief, and mental ability. If you're like most women, exercising is not high on your list of the most pleasurable things to do at 5:30 a.m. before launching into a busy day, or at 8:00 p.m., when your day is winding to a close. Exercise takes time and energy, commodities that are in short supply in our fast-paced, chock-full lives.

Unless you've been holed up in a cave somewhere, you are aware of the benefits of physical activity. I have worked with thousands of clients, helping them get started with exercise. I have also experienced firsthand what it's like to stop and restart an exercise program. It's safe to say that it's a heck of a lot easier to stop than to restart! Just as a reminder of all the great things regular exercise can do for you, let's review its benefits:

▶ Fat loss, especially around the middle

▶ Increased energy all day

▶ Accelerated fat burning for hours even after exercise is over

▶ Enhanced mental concentration and memory

▶ Emotional well-being

▶ Improved self-image

▶ Improved skin tone

▶ Reduced risk for heart disease (30 to 40 percent)

▶ Slowed bone loss and reduced risk for osteoporosis

▶ Improved strength and balance

▶ Improved chronic conditions, such as fibromyalgia (muscle pain) and fatigue

▶ Increased size and tone of your muscles

▶ Revved-up sex drive

▶ Improved outlook on life

▶ Enhanced relationships with those around you

▶ Significantly more efficient weight loss

▶ Reduction in all types of cancer

▶ Hormonal balance!

Inspired? Exercise provides so many direct, measurable benefits that even women who think they don't have a minute to spare should consider re-arranging their priorities. Even if you're not ready to run a marathon just yet, I urge you to choose an activity you enjoy and commit some time each day. Start small—even 20 minutes of walking helps. Take a spinning class or buy a workout videotape. Do it for yourself—and perhaps with a friend! The buddy system is a great motivator.

When it comes to making changes in your life, be realistic. I know we live in a society that says go, go, go and expects instant gratification, but you would be amazed at what you can achieve by changing just one or two habits or activities now and adding something new in a couple of weeks. If you stick with small changes and realistic expectations, within a year it is likely that you will be at or near your goal. When asked about your transformation, you can smile and say that it was just one small step at a time.

Chapter 6

Eliminate the Stress Hormone

IN THIS CHAPTER:

The Story of Stress

The Overworked Adrenal Glands

Where Things Go Wrong for the Busy Woman

Signs of Toxic Stress

Solutions for Resolving Toxic Stress

Diet for Toxic Stress

Exercise for Toxic Stress

We live in an emotionally toxic society that expects women to achieve more and be more in less time. Many of us lead frenzied lives, trying to cram work, exercise, and good nutrition into the same too-brief twenty-four hours—all while trying to be ideal wives and mothers. At the same time, we are expected to be productive, even-tempered, nurturing, libidinous, and, above all, *happy!* If you know a woman who can easily handle the stresses of job, family, and personal upkeep, please let me know; I would like to test her hormones and patent the formula by which she operates!

Most women simply can't handle the overload. During the past decade of treating women, I have noted a pattern in the thirty-five- to fifty-year-old age group. Changes are occurring in these women's physical, emotional, and mental health, and they report significant complaints, including fatigue, depression, PMS, weight gain, repeated flu-like symptoms, cravings, anger, and just not feeling well. I have wondered, *What is this? Why do these outwardly healthy, successful women who have had great energy all of their lives get sucked into a hormonal hurricane?*

The Story of Stress

By the time they come to my office, most women have already seen medical specialists, who had run myriad tests to determine the cause of their fatigue or other medical complaints. When I see them, they are burned out on the medical-office scene and desperate for answers. Most have been advised to seek counseling or psychiatric evaluation, after having been informed that there were no medical problems to treat. Perhaps you've heard that worn-out it's-all-in-your-head diagnosis.

With their all-too-real symptoms continuing unabated, these women commonly ask: "Am I in menopause?" "Could my problems be hormonal?" "Is it stress?" I have to hand it to women: They usually know what's going on with their own bodies. In fact, I have learned to ask women what *they* think is causing their misery, and many times they are right.

It may be difficult to imagine that stress can be a factor in making you fat, initiating depression, and causing hormonal upheaval—but believe it. I have seen it time and again, and stress-related illness is well documented. It is estimated that 43 percent of adults suffer stress-related problems and that 75 to 90 percent of visits to doctors' offices are for stress-related illness. According to Candace Pert, Ph.D., in her book *Molecules of Emotion,* cancer patients' recoveries are significantly slower when anger or emotions are held in, and much research on this phenomenon is being conducted. It has also been well documented that more heart attacks occur on Monday mornings (when the stressful work week begins) than on any other day.

Women are particularly vulnerable to excessive, toxic stress. Taking on more than we should, and not realizing it until it's too late, is often the problem. Many women simply do not recognize the extreme level at which stress is beating them up. It is interesting to note that some of the most healthy, happy women I have ever met are ones who have said no to most of the things you and I would never dream of saying no to. I love questioning these women about how they take care of themselves and why they made the choices they did for their lives. It is also of interest to me that the women with the greatest hormonal upheavals are the ones whose lives are overloaded with stress.

What is most frightening is that the vast majority of women who suffer from excessive toxic stress are the ones who do not recognize that it's stress that is making them sick. Every day, I work with women whom I beg to let go of certain things to have more peace and calmness in their lives and to recapture their health. I have found that many times women will not relinquish the very thing that is making them feel horrible, too often making comments like, "I just can't let go of these things I am responsible for; it would just be too hard." Who says you can't? Who says you have to do everything you are doing? Why can't you say no? Who ultimately pays for your stress? Are you doing the things that really matter? Can you eliminate some things that really don't matter in the big picture?

The Overworked Adrenal Glands

The body is wonderfully wired to respond to emotional, physical, and mental stress. A little danger comes along—such as a truck about to plow into you, a dog rushing to attack, or a 9 a.m. presentation for which you are unprepared—and the adrenal hormones throw on their flak jackets and jump into the bloodstream. Your heart rate accelerates, your blood pressure rises, and blood flow increases to active muscles while decreasing to internal organs. Although this fight-or-flight response is essential to survival in genuine crisis, when it's an everyday occurrence the body's hormonal balance can be sent into a tailspin.

Adrenal hormones have numerous functions in addition to the well-known fight-or-flight response. Located on the tops of the kidneys, the adrenal glands also produce hormones that exert a profound influence on the body's carbohydrate, protein, and fat metabolism; the immune response; thyroid function; cardiovascular health; and overall resistance to stress.

These hormones regulate such vital elements as blood sugar, brain function, muscle use, fluid and electrolyte balance, and more. You don't want to mess with them! When adrenal hormones get out of sync, the immune system is overtaxed; you're less able to cope with stress and more vulnerable to a wide range of illnesses. We're equipped to handle stress. What we were not equipped to handle is the hardcore mental, physical, and emotional loads that so many women endure just to get through the day. Women with un-resolved emotional issues such as continuing conflict, anger, fear, anxiety, and worry bear additional burdens.

Where Things Go Wrong for the Busy Woman

Consider a day in the life of a typical working wife and mother. She gets up too late to exercise and jumps into the shower after yelling at her children to get out of bed. She throws together breakfast for the kids and slaps peanut butter on bread for their lunches. She grabs a cup of coffee and a toaster-pastry for herself while bolting out the door. The gas tank registers empty, and there's no time to fill it. Her workday has meetings scheduled back-to-back, and the kids must be picked up right after work. She knows from the get-go that she'll never get it all done. At about 10 a.m. she takes a few deep breaths and stretches her neck. There's no time for lunch, so she buys snacks from the office vending machine and drinks more coffee. She forgets to drink water. Her workday ends with an overflowing in-box and unanswered messages in her voice-mail box, including one from her best friend, whom she hasn't seen in months. She has no time for friends.

Some co-workers remain at work to finish projects—they're the ones who are headed for promotions—but at 5 p.m. she rushes out to pick up the kids. There's still no gas in the car, so she detours several blocks to a gas station. En route she glares at the ignorant drivers who go the speed limit in no-passing zones. She snaps impatiently at the dawdling gas station attendant before peeling out toward after-school care. A childcare worker taps her watch as our harried mother roars up 15 minutes late. The kids are tired and cranky. She tells herself, *Hang on—you can make it.* She's hungry, tired, and sad, and her thoughts drift to the unopened package of chocolate cookies in the treat drawer at home.

Her husband is home from work and watching TV. "What's for dinner?" he asks, as she flies through the front door. She has no idea and rummages through cupboards and the fridge while chowing down on a cookie. The kids are agitating for food, and one needs help with a science project. Her husband goes for a run.

The mail remains unopened, the laundry basket is full, and the house is a disaster. She settles on macaroni and cheese with wieners, garlic bread, and frozen veggies for dinner. She fills up on the casserole and bread, but has room for ice cream later. She helps one kid with homework while instructing another in the art of washing machine operation. She tucks the kids into bed a half-hour past bedtime, then collapses into bed herself. Her husband insinuates that this would be a great night for sex and edges closer. She groans, but not with pleasure.

If you can relate to any of the above, welcome to the club: You are most likely churning out a poisonous level of stress hormones—a condition I call *toxic stress,* and it's simply too much to withstand on a day-to-day basis. Figure 6-1 recaps the scenario of the working mom and highlights what was happening with this woman's body throughout the day.

Figure 6-1   A day in a life with toxic stress

Event	Consequence
No exercise	Weight gain; no mental, emotional, or physical release for stress management.
Waking up late	Excited, stress response, increasing heart rate and blood pressure.
Poor breakfast	Low blood sugar, which causes her to be tired, irritable, and mentally slow. The caffeine in the coffee overstimulates the nervous system, heightening the stress response.
Rushing the kids	Heightens both the kids' stress response and her own—with guilt.
No preparation	Stress hormones in the blood rise as she rushes to work with no gas and no plan for lunch; knowing that her schedule is too full, anxiety builds.
Inadequate breathing	Stress response heightens with no release; brain gets less oxygen, affecting memory and concentration and causing headaches.
Poor, rushed lunch	Plummeted blood-sugar levels rise abruptly due to the high-sugar carbohydrates consumed with yet another caffeine drink; this causes high insulin levels that result in fat storage, fatigue, irritability, and more cravings.
No time to recover	Days that are overscheduled allow no time to recuperate from stress-hormone overload; mental exhaustion and depression set in.
No time for friends	No laughing, communication, or networking. Recent studies show that women friends help counter stress and are a source of strength and comfort.
Rush after work	Irritation and stress accumulate, prompting an irritable response to strangers.
No help at home	She feels anger, resentment, and irritability and asks herself, *Am I the only one who works around here?* This further increases stress hormones, causing more fat storage, brain fatigue, physical exhaustion, memory loss, and immunity suppression.
Loss of sex drive	No female can thoroughly enjoy sex after a day like this. Apart from her husband's boorish behavior, her mental and physical fatigue contribute to the loss of sex drive.

Solutions for the Stressed-out Busy Woman

Five simple actions could have made all of the difference for this harried woman:

Eating breakfast Include protein at breakfast, then eat at least every four to five hours to maintain blood-sugar levels.

Getting up earlier Go to bed earlier the night before and allow time in the morning to prepare for the day. Taking time to mentally and spiritually brace yourself for what's ahead will quiet the stress response and give you a sense of control.

Exercising If you are unable to get up earlier, try fitting in twenty minutes of walking, playing with the kids, riding your bike, or gentle stretching at some point during the day (see also "Exercise for Toxic Stress" on page 86). Regular exercise offers other benefits as well. An American Cancer Society study in 2001 (published in *Cancer Epidemiology Biomarkers Prevention*) found that women who exercised more than four hours each week had a 37 percent lower breast cancer risk than women who did not exercise.

Relaxing for ten minutes during the day Find a place where when no one can interrupt you. Take time to breathe and quiet yourself to regroup mentally and emotionally. Even a short breather can reduce stress hormone levels.

Nurturing friendship Making time for your friends has a grounding effect, providing nonpressured space to unwind and connect on a healing level.

Signs of Toxic Stress

If you think you are burned out by toxic stress, you probably are. The good news is that you can regain balance and put an end to the hormonal turmoil. It all comes down to self-care. First let's identify the symptoms of toxic stress, which are listed in figure 6-2.

I realize that many readers will check *all* of the symptoms in the figure— I know I have in the past. But I promise that you can gain control over these issues if you are willing to make some positive changes.

Solutions for Resolving Toxic Stress

This section outlines a number of ways to help compensate for the increased levels of stress hormones in your system. Pick and choose what best fits your life. If you are employed, select from both the working-woman list and the

Figure 6-2 Symptoms of toxic stress

Check the ones you have now or have had recently:

☐ Fatigue

☐ Difficult time waking in the morning

☐ Dragging feeling in the afternoon

☐ Poor exercise tolerance

☐ Decreased sex drive

☐ Inability to sleep well, insomnia

☐ Blood sugar fluctuations or hypoglycemia

☐ Increased PMS

☐ Mild to moderate depression

☐ Concerns about menopause

☐ Oversensitivity and criticalness

☐ Impulsiveness

☐ Overreaction to small irritations

☐ Don't-touch-me attitude

☐ Compulsive behaviors

☐ Insatiable appetite

☐ Cravings for sweets or breads

☐ Food binges

☐ Weight gain especially in the middle of your body

general-solutions list. Working women especially need to pay very close attention to their stress level and will need to work harder at guarding their bodies and minds against overload.

Solutions for the Working Woman

▶ **Eat a balanced breakfast every single day.** Include protein. For convenience, try a high-protein bar or breakfast shake. This will help with daily concentration in the workplace and can prevent afternoon fatigue.

▶ **Exercise daily or at least four times per week.** Try to break a sweat each time, but take care not to overexert. Even a lunchtime walk with a co-worker can be a good midday energy boost.

▶ **Plan a recreational activity once a week.** Recreation relieves stress and is a great way to get your body moving and take your mind off workplace or home issues that may be troublesome. Meeting a friend for a Sunday hike with the kids is a great way to catch up, work out, and have a good time.

▶ **Set aside a personal time.** Take *at least* 10 minutes every day. Whether it's soaking in a hot bath or puttering in your yard in the evening, a little time for yourself will always give you a mental boost. Explain the concept of personal time to your kids and teach them to respect it.

Supplements for Stress Management

Supplements can be useful in treating adrenal overload or fatigue. I recommend taking one of the following supplements for four to six weeks and testing its effect on your overall well-being. If you feel better but could use more support, add another supplement.

Licorice root   This is a support supplement for the adrenal glands. Licorice root extract stimulates production and utilization of adrenal hormones.

B-complex   The B vitamins are known as the "stress vitamin" group, as they help the body physically cope with stress. Take a combination, preferably sublingually (see appendix B for guidelines).

Zinc   Try to get at least 30 mg daily. In some cases additional amounts will be needed. Zinc is a natural aromatase enzyme inhibitor that will help create a better balance between estrogen and testosterone, which can become erratic with prolonged stress.

Adrenal support supplements   These are combination botanicals that support adrenal functioning and can be found at health food stores.

Calcium-magnesium supplements   This combination, preferably taken in the evening or before bed, has been shown to promote better sleep, enhance muscle relaxation, increase fat metabolism, and, at doses of 1,000 to 1,200 mg of calcium, boost emotional support.

Phytoestrogens   Consume at least 120 mg of soy isoflavone per day. High levels of isoflavone compete with estradiol on the cell receptor sites and stimulate the liver to remove excessive estrogens from the blood.

▶ **Learn to say no.** Say no whenever saying yes would stretch you too far. Then let it go.

▶ **Take vacations.** A big annual vacation or several short, weekend trips gets your nose away from the grindstone and helps you reconnect with your family on another level. A change of scenery is always refreshing.

▶ **Take mental breaks.** Schedule some deliberate downtime at least once per month—a day or two with few or, if possible, no demands.

▶ **Reserve one day a week for rest, relaxation, and worship.** This is very important. Use this time for self-affirmation and spiritual regrouping. Whether it's meditation, inspirational reading, or attending church services, make time for whatever it is that nurtures your soul.

▶ **Stop listening to negative talk.** Your emotions don't need the stress. Ignore gossip and pettiness that make you feel frustrated or angry.

▶ **Be self-supportive.** Tell yourself you are "worth it" every day—and stop feeling guilty.

▶ **Nurture your friendships.** Have lunch with a friend once a week and do not talk about work.

▶ **Make your workplace positive.** Try to keep your work environment un-cluttered and peaceful.

▶ **Leave your work at the office.** Use the drive home to "change gears" between work mode and personal life. Making a conscious effort to "decompress" will help you clock out mentally as well as physically and keep you from becoming obsessed with your job.

▶ **Practice breathing exercises.** Five times during the day, close your eyes, sit up straight, and breathe in and out through your nose to the count of ten. The calming effect is instant.

Choose at least four things from this list and put them to work in your life. Realize that you are worth the time required for any and all of these stress relievers. You will soon find that such a "sacrifice" becomes a saving grace; the benefits in your life will mount, and the noticeable improvements will be all the incentive you need to keep up the good work.

General Solutions for Every Woman

▶ Take a 30- or 40-minute walk.

▶ Keep a journal of your feelings.

▶ Water your flowers and plants or start a garden.

▶ Clean out your closets or kitchen cabinets, or simply organize a small mess that's been bugging you.

▶ Take a long drive in the country and enjoy the beauty.

▶ Take a trip to the beach and listen carefully to the waves (this one is my favorite).

▶ Enroll in a class just for fun or to develop a new hobby.

▶ Start a new sport or resume an old one.

▶ Learn a craft.

▶ Invite a friend for tea or dinner.

▶ Call a friend who usually energizes you.

▶ Take an inventory of friends and attempt to identify those who energize you and those who drain you. Limit your exposure to the ones who are a strain.

▶ Cry hard and long, if necessary. This is a great release.

▶ Go antique shopping or hit some garage sales.

▶ Attend a religious service or become involved in a church or worship group.

▶ Sleep in or take a nap at least twice a week.

▶ Write a letter to a friend or develop a new friendship.

▶ Take a bath when the family has settled down in the evening—and put a *Do Not Enter* sign on the door.

▶ Get a massage, a facial, or some other self-care treatment.

▶ Read a book.

▶ Meditate.

▶ Pray.

Diet for Toxic Stress

Proper diet is vital as you work your way out of toxic stress. Choose at least three of the dietary guidelines listed below and work toward implementing them into your lifestyle. Even if you're successful at following them just 75 percent of the time, you'll notice improvements.

▶ Drink at least eight to ten glasses of water a day.

▶ Add veggies, protein, and fruit to every meal.

▶ Reduce sugar and refined flour, and eat more whole or sprouted grains. Reducing carbohydrates that have a high sugar release (such as those found in white flour or sugar) and eating a better carbohydrate mix (such as whole grains or sprouted breads) will provide more fiber and less sugar and will help stabilize blood sugar. In addition, complex carbohydrates such as those in whole grains are more satisfying, so you won't feel hungry so soon after eating.

▶ Eat every four to five hours to keep your engine running more smoothly. Providing a steady stream of high-quality fuel will help prevent the blood-sugar fluctuations that lead to cravings and fatigue.

▶ Do not eat sugar, flour, or milk products (such as ice cream) or excessively salty foods near bedtime. If you need to eat them during the day, consume protein first to help stabilize blood sugar.

▶ Keep energy/protein bars or shakes handy at the office for a quick fix when healthy snacks are not on hand. Make sure the energy bars have fewer than 10 grams of sugar and that the protein content is at least 14 grams.

▶ Reduce or eliminate your intake of alcohol and caffeine, which tax the liver where hormones are excreted. Caffeine also overstimulates the nervous system, heightening the stress response, and it is toxic to the liver. Try to limit your consumption of caffeinated beverages to one or two a day, staying below the 200 mg mark on caffeine.

These strategies are essential for creating the right kind of fuel for optimal metabolism. Don't expect your body to perform well if you are feeding it junk. A poor diet will eventually lead to burn-out and long-term health problems. See also chapter 5, "Fix Your Diet: The Most Powerful Way to Create Hormonal Balance."

The Quick-Fix Plan for Stress

Here is an easy-to-follow, quick-fix plan that can be implemented simply and immediately with dramatic effects.

Breathe Take ten deep breaths in and out at least twice daily. When you feel stress climbing, close your eyes and concentrate on slow and controlled breathing. Breathe in through your nose to the count of four and breathe out to the count of six or seven. Repeat 10 times. You will feel better!

Eat at regular intervals Include protein in your diet as well as plenty of whole grains, fruits, and veggies. Avoid fast food and other sugary, fat-laden foods.

Stay hydrated Drink at least eight glasses of water a day.

Exercise Daily exercise promotes good health physically, mentally, and emotionally—and you'll look better too!

Pamper yourself Take daily time-outs. When you do this, the stress hormones have nowhere to go but down. Focusing on yourself for even a few minutes will provide a break from the intensity and allow your adrenals a much-needed rest. The mental boost you gain from taking a break better equips you to deal with the sources of stress.

Laugh, pray, and smile And tell yourself you are worth being blessed.

Exercise for Toxic Stress

▶ Include low-impact, medium-intensity workouts such as brisk walking, cycling, or a step class at least three times weekly—but don't overdo it. Pushing your body with adrenal fatigue or excessive stress will only make the situation worse.

▶ Exercise that increases strength and flexibility, such as Pilates, will complement your stress management plan. They're easy to do at home and require little time and equipment.

Sources of stress are not going to disappear, so how you choose to handle stress or alleviate it is the key. If you take steps today to reduce the effects of stress in your life, you'll reap a host of positive outcomes; these can include increased energy, fewer cravings, reduction in body fat, less irritability and depression, and most likely an improved sense of well-being. In addition, you will begin steering away from such stress-related afflictions as memory loss, difficulty concentrating, muscle fatigue, depression, and weight gain.

Chapter 7

Get a Grip on PMS

IN THIS CHAPTER:

PMS During Perimenopause

What Causes PMS?

Diagnosing PMS

PMS Treatment Options

Jenny is often depressed, nervous, and angry without knowing why. She screams at her kids, expects her husband to read her mind, and becomes agitated and angry over minor irritations. *Why do I blow things out of proportion?* she asks herself. She concludes that, like the other women in her family, she is an irritable, moody person and that it is simply beyond her control. But deep in her guilt-ridden heart she believes that if only she had greater inner strength, she could gain power over her moods and save the people she loves most from her lashing tongue and foul temper.

Jenny is approaching forty and realizes with alarm that her symptoms now occur most of the month, not just during the few days before her period, as they did when she was younger. It used to be as though someone flipped on a switch a week or so before her period, and she turned into a shrew. Then her period would arrive, and she'd mellow out until the next month, when the switch was flipped again.

But things have gotten worse, and now the switch is nearly always on. The only time she feels like a normal, warm-hearted human being is during the week she is actually menstruating. Looking back, she connects her lengthening bouts of depression and anger with the arrival of her last child. Following the birth, and a tubal ligation to prevent future pregnancies, her dark moods were even darker and extended from period to period.

Jenny's doctor advises her to reduce stress, improve her nutrition, and use mood-leveling antidepressants. The drugs put her on a more even keel, but they make her feel bloated and tired, so she quits them after just a few months. As for stress, Jenny can't see a solution. She juggles a demanding full-time job outside the home and a demanding full-time job *inside* the home. Her husband and three kids require food, clothing, and attention regardless of what's going on with her emotional life.

Her kids complain about her moods, and her husband insists she needs medication, but her mother reassures her that she's normal—that most of the women in her family have had the same thing. Normal or not, Jenny feels guilty, sad, and out of control.

Jenny, of course, has had classic *premenstrual syndrome (PMS)* for most of her adult life. Any woman who has black-and-white mood swings related to her period is most likely suffering from this common condition.

PMS During Perimenopause

There are more than 150 acknowledged symptoms of PMS, both physical and emotional. Approximately 85 percent of menstruating women have one or more PMS symptoms. Of those women, as many as 10 to 20 percent experience profound symptoms that, as in Jenny's case, cast a dark, unbroken cloud over their lives.

Authors of the book *The Hormone Connection* cite the work of medical researcher Neill Epperson, M.D., professor of psychiatry and obstetrician gynecologist at Yale University, who found that an increased risk of mood disturbance is connected with major hormonal events such as beginning menstruation, giving birth, and starting into menopause. Some 19 million U.S. adults each year struggle with sadness, hopelessness, and major depression. Two-thirds of these are women.

PMS symptoms often include irritability, depression, and fatigue. Other mood-related symptoms include paranoia, anger, sadness, guilt, weepiness, desire to escape, and feelings of worthlessness. The physical symptoms can occur together or singly and include headaches, food cravings, water retention, breast tenderness, acne, hives, cold sores, herpes outbreaks, asthma, throat or gland swelling, seizures, recurrent yeast or bladder infections, and flu-like symptoms. Some women have migraines only before their periods.

What Causes PMS?

PMS cannot be pinned on any one causative factor or even a few factors. Some believe that a diet low in fiber and protein and high in sugar, refined carbo-hydrates, and animal or trans-fats can result in fluctuating blood-sugar and high insulin levels, which lead to depression, erratic moods, bloating, and weight gain. Others believe that a vitamin B_6 deficiency or the imbalanced ratio of calcium to magnesium may be at fault. Some researchers contend that PMS is a hormonal problem resulting from low progesterone or estrogen levels—or both. Some experts in the field of women's health suggest that some women with PMS have low adrenal output of DHEA and other adrenal hormones necessary for stress control.

Yet other researchers conclude that PMS is a neuroendocrin imbalance. This imbalance may take place in the higher centers of the brain and trigger hormones that affect the output of important brain chemicals such as serotonin, norepinephrine, dopamine, and endorphins. In women with PMS, the release of endorphins (the feel-good brain chemicals) may be significantly different than the release in women without PMS. Neuroendocrine research suggests that women with PMS have levels of endorphins that are only 25 percent of those of women who do not suffer from PMS.

In addition, current research indicates that women with PMS may have fewer progesterone receptors. Typically, after women reach thirty-five, ovulation becomes irregular and hormonal balance begins to tip. Katharina Dalton, M.D., a British pioneer who has studied PMS for more than thirty years, suggests that women with PMS have a deficiency in circulating progesterone and that they respond to natural progesterone supplementation during the second half of the menstrual cycle.

Another school of thought hangs the blame for PMS on the ratio of progesterone to estrogen. As women get into the perimenopausal years, ovulation becomes irregular. Progesterone is produced primarily by the ovaries at the time of ovulation (it is also made in small amounts by the adrenal glands). When ovulation fails to occur, progesterone levels drop and estrogen dominates, often resulting in mood swings.

The effects of birth control pills or synthetic progestins on PMS are unclear. Some researchers conclude that the pill and synthetic progestins make women feel more irritable and depressed, whereas others believe that the pill may promote mood stabilization by restoring the estrogen balance.

Doctors Norman Beals Jr. and Norman Beals Sr. have spent more than sixty combined years studying PMS and other female hormonal changes. Their clinical investigation of women suffering from PMS would point to lowered progesterone levels in the second half of the menstrual cycle. Other researchers in the area of PMS have shown a beneficial effect with using progesterone in treatment of PMS. Research published by R. V. Norris in the *Journal of Reproductive Medicine* on the use of progesterone for premenstrual tension found it to be a safe, useful, and effective treatment for severe PMS.

I have long been struck by the frequent and repetitive pattern of mood changes that women experience the closer they get to menopause. It is fascinating to see women whom I have known for years as emotionally balanced human beings completely fall apart prior to their periods once they reach their thirties and forties. For many women hormonal upheaval is compounded by having to juggle schedules while managing homes, families, and businesses.

With respect to mood changes and PMS in my patients, I see the following patterns as women age:

▶ PMS worsens in the late thirties.

▶ In their late thirties and early forties, most women have low circulating levels of progesterone (the mood hormone).

▶ The late thirties and forties are typically the time during which patients start requesting prescriptions for antidepressants.

▶ Women gain weight much easier after the age of thirty-five, causing depression and lack of self-esteem.

▶ Midlife depression can often be reduced or turned around completely with lifestyle changes and hormone balancing.

In her book *Screaming to Be Heard,* Elizabeth Lee Vliet, M.D., notes that a variety of studies in recent years have demonstrated that neuroreceptors respond to circulating hormones of all kinds, including the female hormones estradiol, progesterone, and testosterone. This means that brain chemicals are positively and negatively affected by high and low hormone levels. Both brain and body have multitudes of these sensitive hormone receptors. Dr. Vliet also observes that changes in estrogen, progesterone, and testosterone during the perimenopausal years have significant effects on the brain chemicals dopamine, norepinephrine, acetylcholine, and serotonin—all powerful mood modulators.

Factors Increasing the Incidence and Severity of PMS

Childbirth   The more births, the more severe the PMS.

Tubal ligation   Although not researched or documented in the literature, I have seen an overwhelming number of women who have had a tubal ligation go on to suffer significant PMS symptoms that they did not have prior to the surgery.

Age   PMS increases with age. Women in their thirties are most prone to developing PMS.

Stress   Exposure to stress worsens PMS.

Diet   High intake of caffeine, refined sugar, salt, and excessive refined carbohydrates as well as poor eating habits such as skipping meals or overeating worsen PMS.

Physical activity   Lack of exercise worsens PMS.

Diagnosing PMS

If symptoms occur regularly and are related to the menstrual cycle, PMS is likely. Symptoms generally appear during the week or two before menstruation begins and end abruptly once bleeding starts. It is a good idea to keep a diary of your menstrual cycle for at least three months. Note your symptoms, their severity, and when they occur. When you visit your doctor, this information will be very useful for arriving at a diagnosis and a treatment plan.

Because PMS may be present for many days each month and has some symptoms similar to menopause, it can be confused with menopause. If the symptoms persist throughout the month, other conditions to consider, in addition to menopause, include thyroid deficiency, anemia, adrenal fatigue, or a combination thereof.

PMS Assessment

The checklist in figure 7-1 can help you determine whether you suffer from PMS, depression, or other mood disorders. I use this assessment in my office to help women pinpoint their feelings and define their symptoms. It is also used as a baseline for comparison once treatment has been started.

Figure 7-1   PMS assessment checklist

1. Do you experience the following mood changes?

	Before Period	2 to 3 Weeks per Month	All Month
Anger	☐	☐	☐
Irritability	☐	☐	☐
Depression	☐	☐	☐
Erratic moods	☐	☐	☐
Rage	☐	☐	☐
Crying spells	☐	☐	☐

2. Do you experience the following physical changes?

☐ Weight gain	☐ Hands/feet swelling
☐ Breast tenderness	☐ Dry skin
☐ Hair loss	☐ Headaches
☐ Low-back pain	☐ Hot flashes
☐ Ovarian pain	☐ Constipation

3. Do you experience the following in your behavior?

☐ Increased cravings	☐ Insomnia
☐ Fatigue	☐ Lack of coordination
☐ Forgetfulness	☐ Indecision

If you experience at least four of the symptoms listed in figure 7-1 and have them prior to your period, you are suffering from PMS. If you experience ten or more, it is likely that PMS is significantly altering your life. The number of days during which you are affected is also important. If you have symptoms more than five days per month, you need to seek testing and treatment. If you experience these symptoms continuously without relief, I would recommend getting a comprehensive hormone profile and a general health evaluation without delay. This would include additional testing for blood sugar, thyroid, iron levels, and possibly depression. If your symptoms significantly interrupt your life and compromise your overall well-being, consider the following suggestions.

PMS Treatment Options

Steps You Can Take on Your Own

Even before you see your healthcare provider, some simple actions and lifestyle changes may help ease your symptoms.

Seek support   Acknowledge the significance of PMS, especially to those close to you, and involve them in your efforts for relief. Explain what you're going through, and ask for support in trying to reduce stressors during the "bad" days of the month.

Reduce stress   Evaluate the stressors in your life, and try to minimize stressful situations and exposure to negative personality types. Eliminate things that you do not need to be dealing with, even if it means letting go of responsibilities.

Get moving   Increase your outdoor activities and exercise. Regular exercise can have a profound effect on mood and overall health. Develop a daily plan for getting fresh air and working your body through exercise—and stick to it. You can't expect to feel balanced and well if you work your head all week at the office but neglect to work your body. The buddy system is a great motivator for keeping to an exercise regimen.

Pay attention to diet   The hypoglycemia diet works best for treating high and low moods and seesawing energy levels. (See "Guidelines for the Hypoglycemia Diet" on page 94.) Women who have sudden attacks of irritability can also benefit from this style of eating, as their blood-sugar levels can fluctuate erratically. Dietary supplements can help, too (see "Supplements" on page 94).

Adding chocolate to the diet can help. Really! This happens to be my favorite treatment for PMS. Chocolate (the real thing) can increase serotonin levels in the brain, which ultimately improves mood. Real chocolate also contains theobromine, which is similar to caffeine and can temporarily boost energy. I suggest savoring a couple pieces of good chocolate prior to the period. Pay attention to the amount because, unfortunately, chocolate is approximately 50 percent fat and 50 percent sugar.

If bloating is a problem, natural or prescribed diuretics can help. Both over-the-counter condensed cranberry tablets and prescription spironolactone are effective. Spironolactone is the most beneficial mild diuretic and has effects

Guidelines for the Hypoglycemia Diet

■ Eat small, frequent meals.

■ Combine protein with each meal or snack.

■ Eliminate alcohol, caffeine, and artificial colorings.

■ Do not eat sugar or flour-starchy foods on an empty stomach. Eat protein first to stabilize the blood sugar.

■ Eat four to six servings of fruit and vegetables daily.

It is also a good idea to restrict salt, which can cause excessive water retention before periods, and avoid alcohol. Drinking alcohol causes blood-sugar fluctuations and tends to produce irritability when the blood-sugar level drops.

similar to progesterone. It can also help with reducing acne and facial hair. Many natural diuretics are also available as herbal teas.

Supplements

Evening primrose oil (EPO) capsules   Several studies have shown the effectiveness of EPO in treating PMS. EPO contains an essential fatty acid that helps promote a prostaglandin that inhibits the action of prolactin. Prolactin is found in high levels in women with PMS and can cause progesterone levels to drop. The use of EPO can help reverse this process and promote well-being. It is also helpful for menstrual cramps and heavy bleeding. The typical dose is 500 to 1,200 mg per day.

Vitamin D with calcium and magnesium   Calcium and magnesium can significantly aid in sleep when taken in the evening. Several recent studies have shown an improvement in PMS symptoms with the use of calcium supplements. Vitamin D has been shown to have a positive effect in regulating energy metabolism and completely reversing PMS.

The typical dose is 500 to 1,200 mg of calcium with magnesium daily. In our office we use a liquid cal/mag that is extremely well absorbed and helpful for symptom relief.

B-Complex   B-complex is a "stress vitamin complex" that can help improve the body's response to stress by relieving cravings as well as joint and muscle pain and by increasing energy, memory, and mental concentration.

The typical dose is 1,000 mcg of B_{12} or B-100 complex. In my office we use a sublingual preparation that is adequately absorbed and is an excellent PMS pickup.

Herbs   Herbal supplements such as licorice root, wild yam root, astragalus, dong quai, ginger, vitex, burdock root, motherwort, horsetail, and red clover can be helpful in treating PMS. I suggest an herbal combination of some of these in a tincture form that is fresh and of high grade. (See "Vitamin and Herbal Supplements" in appendix B.)

L-tyrosine   This amino acid can be extremely helpful in alleviating depression and low moods. It should be started in low doses and used regularly for two months to evaluate the effects.

5-HTP   The typical dose is 50 to 100 mg once or twice daily to improve the mood and provide excellent sleep quality.

Progesterone Therapy

Without a doubt progesterone therapy is a godsend to women. I can honestly say *it just works!* The majority of women I see for depression and PMS have low circulating levels of progesterone. It is interesting to note that PMS most often occurs in the second half of the menstrual cycle, which is when progesterone levels are supposed to be highest.

Before prescribing progesterone, or in some cases, estrogen, it is necessary to test the levels in the blood. Of utmost importance, the testing should be done during the luteal phase of the cycle, which is the second half of the cycle, when progesterone is being secreted during ovulation. It has been noted that with increasing age, however, ovulation becomes irregular.

Natural progesterone absorbs well through the skin, as do many other hormones and medications. It can also be prescribed as a sublingual lozenge, a tablet, a capsule, drops, or a vaginal suppository. I recommend taking progesterone from day 14 of the cycle to day 28. Some women need to start early in the month, as their symptoms begin between days 7 and 10. It is important to use the progesterone faithfully so that irregular bleeding does not occur. (See also "Recommended Options for Progesterone Therapy" on page 96.)

Recommended Options for Progesterone Therapy

Progesterone capsules The typical dose is 100 mg taken once or twice daily. The capsules can be formulated by a trained pharmacist to provide a true sustained release throughout the day, allowing for fewer side effects.

Progesterone drops or lozenges (under the tongue) The typical dose is 50 to 100 mg once or twice daily for symptom relief.

Progesterone creams/gels (topical on the skin) Rub 20 to 60 mg into the skin once or twice daily. Both over-the-counter and prescription doses are taken in the amount that relieves symptoms. Apply the cream to thin-skinned areas, such as the inner arms, breasts, neck, face, brows, or inner thighs. I have found that most women do better on a higher-dose (3 to 10 percent) prescription cream rather than an over-the-counter preparation, which is a 1.5 to 3 percent cream. As some women experience sleepiness when using progesterone, a smaller dose is often used in the morning.

Est-Pro The typical dose is 0.35 mg micronized estradiol with 100 mg micronized progesterone in an oil base—one capsule one to two times daily. This is a combination of natural estrogen and progesterone in a capsule form.

Estrogen A low-dose estrogen patch in combination with progesterone one to two weeks before the period can provide excellent sleep, a reduction in hot flashes, mood control, and increased energy.

Antidepressants

Antidepressants are definitely not my first line of treatment. I believe that the majority of PMS symptoms can be dramatically improved with diet, supplements, exercise, and, if relief is not evident, hormone therapy. Prescription antidepressants, however, are an option for women who have tried everything and are still suffering from severe emotional symptoms. Antidepressant drugs such as Prozac do not relieve physical PMS symptoms.

If you believe that your mood disorder goes beyond PMS, I recommend that you seek help for depression and mood instability. In addition, request a hormone evaluation at two different times in your cycle for comparison. Hormonal imbalance can wreak havoc on your mental and physical health.

Whatever you do, if you are suffering from PMS and it is only getting worse with age, don't delay trying the suggestions in this chapter. Why wait when you can feel better now?

Chapter 8

Turn on Your Sex Drive

IN THIS CHAPTER:

Is Losing Libido Inevitable?

What Is a "Healthy" Sex Drive?

Hormones to Increase Sex Drive

Alternatives for Improving Sex Drive

Additional Sex-Drive Blasters

If it wasn't for ruining her marriage, it would have been fine with Kate if she never had sex again. She was tired, overweight, frustrated, and just not at all interested. In fact, the very thought of going through the act made her cringe. Of course, Kate felt guilty. She didn't want to let her husband down with her lack of enthusiasm, but she just couldn't fake it. She had a hectic schedule and was tired of trying to make everyone around her feel great; it seemed as though she was the only one who didn't benefit from her forced good cheer. Sex was the one area where she drew the line—even though she missed the closeness that a good sex life brings to a relationship—and her husband was becoming more distant with each refusal.

Kate knew she had to deal with her complete lack of libido—but how? When she came to my office, I asked if she was *really* ready to work on her sex life. After a marginal commitment, she agreed to begin. The initial evaluation included hormone tests, a physical exam, a stress evaluation, and a review of lovemaking practices and relationship issues.

Blood tests showed that Kate had marginally low levels of both female testosterone and DHEA; she agreed to try a small dose of testosterone gel with a DHEA supplement daily for three months. She also had vaginal dryness and irritation, for which I prescribed a hormonal combination cream.

Kate agreed to tell her partner that she wanted to work on their sex life and to ask for his help and commitment. With his cooperation, she started one hour of relaxation before bed on two designated nights per week. During this time her partner was in charge of the household, while she lounged in the bath with candles and aromatherapy. She talked more openly to her husband about what she enjoyed sexually and made a conscious effort to have sensual thoughts about him early in the day that she planned to have sex.

What Kate discovered is *the more you have sex, the more you want it.* This is true for all men and women. Hormones necessary for a healthy sex life are released when you have sex, so the greater the frequency, the greater the desire. Kate also realized that she felt better about herself when she made love twice weekly—and that her husband felt better about her, too. He was kinder to her and was more willing to help with domestic chores, and their relationship grew deeper almost immediately.

After the initial dose of testosterone, Kate no longer needed the supplement but continued with the DHEA, which helped stabilize her hormones. Today she is an avid spokesperson to her friends about the importance of having a good sex life.

Is Losing Libido Inevitable?

If you are in your late thirties or forties and your libido is in the tank, rest assured that you are not alone! Loss of sexual desire is all too common. I see women every day who are frustrated, depressed, and guilt-ridden over the fact that they have lost interest in hopping into the sack.

If the sex thing weren't so emotionally charged, it would be much easier to manage. Men, whose testosterone keeps them in a state of near-constant sexual readiness, rarely understand when their mates "aren't in the mood." They take it personally and begin to doubt their desirability and manliness. They may seek sexual gratification elsewhere or take out their frustrations in other unpleasant ways. Either way, no sex—or grudging sex—leads to hurt feelings, self-doubt, and tension in a relationship. Both partners lose.

Women with healthy, active sex lives enjoy a rich emotional connection with their mates. Vibrant sexuality pumps them up with vitality and provides the hormone balance needed for harmonious relationships. It is a cruel irony that the less frequently we have sexual intimacy, the less we desire it. On the other hand, the more often we have fulfilling, nurturing, sexual activity, the more sex-drive hormones are released and the greater is our sexual desire. Sex is a prime example of "use it or lose it."

Did You Know…?

- Loss of sexual desire in women in their late thirties or forties is all too common—but it's not a permanent condition.

- The most likely culprit for a lack of libido is hormonal imbalance or deficiency.

- The more often you have sexual activity, the more sex-drive hormones are released and the greater your sexual desire.

- Vibrant sexuality gives you vitality and provides the hormone balance you need for harmonious relationships.

- Testosterone—the "male hormone"—is also produced by the ovaries and the adrenal glands and is a significant factor in creating a normal, healthy sex drive in women.

- Estrogen primes the brain cells for sexual activity, and progesterone helps turn on the libido.

- A woman loses approximately 50 percent of her testosterone between the ages of thirty-five and fifty.

If you suffer from low libido, reduced sexual arousal or sensation, or difficulty achieving orgasm, or if you experience discomfort while having sex, this chapter is for you. I have kept it simple and to the point, with proven tips on how to turn your sex life around.

What Is a "Healthy" Sex Drive?

Let's spend a quick little minute on what creates a sex drive, starting with the basics: sex hormones and the brain. When I say "the brain," I am referring only to the physiological aspects of sex, not all the mental and emotional stuff that gets in the way of women's enjoying it.

The *hypothalamus,* a cherry-sized region of the brain, indirectly controls the release of numerous hormones, including sex hormones. Loss of function in this area can result in, among others things, the loss of appetite for food, sleep, and sex. Because disorders of the hypothalamus are usually caused by a brain hemorrhage or a pituitary tumor, it is unlikely that a hypothalamus disorder is the underlying cause for a sluggish libido. The more likely culprit is hormonal imbalance or deficiency.

Here's something you might not know: Testosterone, the potent hormone produced by male testicles that makes men out of boys, is also produced in

Foods to Fuel the Fire

Prepare some elegant temptations that are high in complex carbohydrates and protein for energy and low in saturated heavy fats so as not to slow you down. The identification of *aphrodisiacs* (foods that enhance sexual desire) dates back some five thousand years. Libido and sexual potency decreases without sufficient nutrients, so the number one rule is to make sure your food is nutrient packed!

- **Chocolate** Probably the most popular of all aphrodisiacs, chocolate possesses a sedative that causes relaxation and lowering of inhibitions that encourages increased activity. Sometimes even just the aroma will result in a release of hormones that increase desire. It also contains cancer-fighting enzymes—but remember that *moderation is the key!*

- **Chilies and cayenne peppers** These capsicums are rich in vitamin C and protein, which is good for circulation to keep the blood pumping.

- **Champagne or wine** A toast with alcohol can help set the celebratory mood, but drink only in moderation—enough to help you relax but not so much as to have a sedative effect.

- **Ginger** This rhizome, considered "the Viagra of food," can increase circulation of blood throughout the body. Use moderately in cooking or choose a ginger dish when eating out.

- **Pineapple** Rich in vitamin C, pineapple is often used to treat impotency.

- **Lobster** Rife with all the necessary ingredients for stimulating the body, lobster contains sulfur, calcium, iron, amino acids, and vitamin B—all necessary for healthy sexual desire.

- **Oysters** These very nutritious mollusks are rich in vitamins and minerals. They are low in fat and high in protein and zinc, which is important for sex drive.

- **Strawberries and raspberries** Often described as "sexual fruits," these berries are loaded with vitamins necessary for circulation and stimulation.

small amounts by the ovaries and the adrenal glands. It is an absolutely essential part of a woman's hormonal brew and a significant factor in a normal, healthy sex drive. A balance of estrogen and progesterone also creates sexual health: Estrogen primes the brain cells for sexual activity, and progesterone is known to help turn on the libido.

Of course, sex drive is also influenced by past experiences, energy level, self-confidence, self-esteem, physical health, relationship issues and feelings toward partner, and emotional well-being. All that aside, hormones are key, especially testosterone.

A woman loses approximately 50 percent of her testosterone between the ages of thirty-five and fifty, but the sorry truth is that many women start experiencing lower testosterone levels much earlier in life. Like all hormones, testosterone can become deficient when we are under stress. The adrenals—our "stress glands"—pump out excess stress hormones when we are chronically tense and anxious, resulting over time in reduced libido and exhaustion.

As women enter the premenopausal years, ages thirty-five to fifty, ovulation becomes irregular and the ovaries secrete less testosterone. At the same time, reduced estrogen can cause thinning of the vaginal lining and external tissues, which can result in painful sex. Fortunately, sexual vitality and zest can often be restored. Jennifer Berman, M.D., director of the Female Sexual Medicine Center at the University of California, Los Angeles, has found that women whose ovaries have been removed have more complaints of loss of feeling in the clitoral area. These women can also experience reduced intensity of orgasm or an inability to achieve orgasm at all. This can be from the loss of ovarian testosterone, or reduced blood flow to the clitoral or labial areas. I have spent time working with Dr. Berman at the UCLA clinic and am encouraged that there is a growing interest in helping women achieve better sexual function. If you suffer from lower sex drive, reduced sexual feeling, inability to achieve orgasm, or painful sex, there are options for you!

Hormones to Increase Sex Drive

The first step toward improving your sex drive is ensuring that you are secure in your relationship with your partner; emotional issues can and do get in the way of sexual desire. The second step is to make sure that your lifestyle is not so demanding that it is physically impossible for you to relax and enjoy sex. This means you are successfully managing stress and that your diet and physical activity are conducive to a healthy sex drive. If everything else seems to be in reasonable order, the third step is to have your hormone levels tested to determine if a prescription for hormone balance is right for you.

This last step, regarding the quality of blood flow to the vaginal, clitoral, and labial tissues, involves an evaluation by your medical provider. The doctor uses an ultrasound specifically designed to monitor the blood flow to the genital tissues. The evaluation can also be done utilizing sensitive equipment aimed at identifying loss of sensation or feeling to the tissues. Although most medical practitioners are not equipped to conduct this type of evaluation, they can also evaluate you through a physical examination and by listening to your medical and sexual history.

An estimated 16 to 20 million women in the United States are deficient in testosterone and experience low libido—and all the emotional baggage that comes with it. Only 5 percent are being helped. Healthcare providers have a responsibility to meet women's needs in this area. Restored sexual desire promotes feelings of overall well-being and leads to hormonal balance, less depression and resentment, improved self-image, and healthier relationships in general.

Hormone Therapy

The following are specific suggestions to guide you to greater sexual desire and satisfaction. Don't hesitate to bring these measures to the attention of your healthcare provider.

Testosterone   If hormone testing reveals your testosterone level to be below the normal range, using a testosterone replacement in female-sized doses can turn your sex life around. Both natural and synthetic testosterone are available, but I strongly recommend the natural type, as the side effects are minimal and the treatment is very effective. Other hormones, including natural progesterone, may also be beneficial.

Synthetic preparations of testosterone such as Estratest and Android contain methyltestosterone, which can have many unwanted side effects. Natural testosterone, or Testosterone USP, is a bioidentical hormone (with the same structure as human testosterone) compounded as a prescription cream, pill, sublingual drop, or lozenge. The natural molecularly identical testosterone replacement not only produces an excellent effect on the sex drive, but also protects against osteoporosis, improves muscle tone and strength, and boosts energy. Susan Rako, M.D., author of *The Hormone Desire: The Truth About Sexuality, Menopause, and Testosterone,* says that evidence is accumulating that testosterone replacement is not only helpful for osteoporosis prevention but also in the treatment of osteoporosis.

The advantages of the transdermal testosterone cream are that it is absorbed through the skin and heads directly for the target tissues and only later passes through the liver, where the hormone is broken down. Glenn D. Braunstein, M.D., chairman of the Department of Medicine at Cedars-Sinai Medical Center in Los Angeles, notes in the *New England Journal of Medicine* that women who undergo ovarian removal or who show signs of testosterone loss in menopause could benefit from testosterone use. It can help ease the transition and improve mood, energy, and libido.

The downside to using testosterone are the side effects if the levels are too high; these include acne, deepened voice, hair growth, and irritability. A small amount such as 0.5 mg (which is twenty-five to thirty times smaller than a man's prescription) can be started initially. Women who start with a daily dose of 0.5 to 4 mg rarely experience unwanted side effects. If side effects do occur, reducing the dose or frequency of use will most likely eliminate them.

Natural progesterone   This bioidentical substance is derived from plant sources. It can be formulated by a compounding pharmacy or sold over-the-counter as a cream. It can also be compounded in a pharmacy by prescription if a higher dose is needed.

DHEA   Sold over-the-counter or as a prescription supplement, DHEA can be added if its level in your blood is low. Taking 10 to 25 mg daily in the morning can increase energy, strength, endurance, and libido while reducing pain and fatigue. DHEA can also be prescribed through a compounding pharmacy to a prescribed dose.

Estradiol   This hormone eases perimenopausal changes and improves hormonal balance. When used vaginally, it can relieve dryness and irritation.

Estriol   When used as a vaginal cream, estriol is excellent for vaginal dryness and thinning. This medication is available only by prescription through a compounding pharmacy.

Alternatives for Improving Sex Drive

There are many things that you can do to kick-start your libido and thereby spice up your love life. The following suggestions can be implemented in addition to hormone therapy, or they can be tried as alternatives to testosterone and/or other hormone prescriptions.

Make some positive lifestyle changes   The bottom line is we feel sexier when we feel better about ourselves. Here are some simple things you can do to feel better in general:

▶ Exercise for 20 to 50 minutes daily or at least three to four times per week. (See "Simple Exercises for Improved Body Image" on page 105.)

▶ Improve your diet by avoiding high-fat foods that make you feel sluggish. A high-fat meal, especially with dessert or alcohol, will cause you to feel tired and unable to perform as you would like. (See chapter 5.)

▶ Take 1 tablespoon of flaxseed oil as a daily supplement.

▶ Increase your daily intake of soy to 30 to 50 g.

▶ Avoid sugar and white flour. Use sprouted-wheat breads, and stay away from packaged cookies and crackers.

▶ Add lean protein to each meal.

Do Kegel exercises daily   Tighten the vaginal muscles (as if you were stopping urination) and hold for a count of 10. Repeat five times, several times daily. You can also order the Kegel Master, a device that strengthens the pelvic muscles to enhance orgasms and reduce incontinence-related problems. (See "Products for Sexual Dysfunction" in appendix C.)

Use a circulation enhancer   If you have lost sensation in the genital area, you may want to consider one of the following for enhanced arousal:

▶ Try the Eros Stimulator for improved sensation. This device is designed to bring blood flow to the area prior to sexual activity. (See "Products for Sexual Dysfunction" in appendix C.)

▶ Try Viagra cream for enhanced sensation. Prescription topical Viagra-like cream or topical testosterone/estriol cream can be obtained from a compounding pharmacy. These are applied to the clitoral area prior to intercourse. (See "Compounding Pharmacies" in appendix A.)

▶ Try topical prescription medications that are aimed at increasing circulation to the genital area. These medications can provide significant improvement in sensation when applied to the clitoral/vaginal area prior to sexual activity.

▶ Ask your doctor about prescription Viagra or a Viagra-like cream that will enhance arousal and sexual stimulation.

Simple Exercises for Improved Body Image

In less than an hour a day, you can make great strides toward more self-esteem while improving your health, longevity, and libido at the same time. In just a few weeks, both you and your partner will notice the physical results, but *do it for yourself!* Once you establish the habit of daily exercise, it becomes second nature, and you'll find yourself *wanting* to exercise—you'll actually miss it if you skip a day!

- *Crunches*—to tighten the tummy. Start with 10 a day, and add 5 or 10 per week until you can do 100. You can do these from a sitting position as well as while lying on your back; each will tighten slightly different abdominals, thus compounding the effects. You'll see results in just a couple of weeks!

- *Side bends,* preferably with small hand weights. Keeping your legs, arms, and back straight, and your shoulders down, bend sideways at the waist. Bend left, straighten, bend right, repeat. You'll be amazed at how quickly this simple movement trims inches from your waist.

- *Overhead triceps extension to tighten undersides of upper arms.* Stand erect with feet shoulder width apart. Holding a soup can in your hand, point your elbow straight up. Raise hand to a 90-degree angle while keeping your elbow still; hold for five counts and repeat. Now do the other arm.

- *Leg lifts* to trim the inner thighs. Lie on your side and lift your top leg up, perpendicular to the floor. Repeat 10 times with toe pointed, then 10 times with foot flexed. Switch sides and do the other leg. Start with 10 a day, and add 5 or 10 per week until you can do 100.

- *Shoulders back, ladies.* This makes you appear pounds thinner than when hunched over, and it builds your upper back and neck muscles at the same time. You'll feel less strain when sitting at a computer after a long day.

Consider light therapy   Light may be a factor affecting your sex drive. Many women suffer from seasonal affective disorder (SAD). If sunlight is not abundant where you live, consider getting a full-spectrum light for your home. (See "Products for Treatment of PMS" in appendix C.)

Use supplements   There are numerous supplements believed to enhance sex drive; these include the following:

- ▶ **L-arginine.** Studies have shown that this amino acid can increase sex drive and sensation. L-arginine can be taken orally, or it can be compounded to be applied topically to the clitoral area for increased sensation.

▶ **Vitamin E.** The typical daily dosage of vitamin E is 200 to 400 IU (international units). This antioxidant not only can help improve libido, but when applied topically to the genital area it can reduce dryness and thinning of tissues. When taken orally it can also reduce perimenopausal symptoms such as hot flashes and night sweats.

▶ **Adrenal and liver support supplements.** These supplements will assist in improving the absorption and excretion of hormones through the liver to enhance overall balance and effect. (See "Getting your liver in shape" in chapter 4.)

Additional Sex-Drive Blasters

This section outlines some additional factors that can put a damper on your love life. Addressing and eliminating any of the following will help fan the flames.

Vaginal dryness   The vaginal lining contains glands that secrete fluid when stimulated by hormones produced by the ovaries. Vaginal dryness is usually caused by the decreased hormone production that can occur during perimenopause. The use of lubricants that can be purchased over-the-counter, such as aloe jelly and vitamin E oil, can help with vaginal dryness.

To reverse chronic dryness, a prescription for estriol vaginal cream applied externally will improve tissue elasticity and make it more youthful and lubricated. The use of 2 percent testosterone gel can also provide excellent recovery of the tissues. Kegel exercises, in which you tighten the vaginal muscles as though you were stopping urination, can help build up the muscles that support the pelvic floor. Kegel exercises also help improve sexual sensation and lubrication naturally.

Poor communication   Discussing your sexual relationship with your partner is imperative to a healthy sex life. Let your partner know what you are feeling emotionally and physically. (Such intimate conversations are usually best conducted *out* of bed.) Reassure your partner that your lack of libido is no reflection on his or her desirability. Such disclosures can be very healing to a stressed relationship. Including your partner in your efforts to rekindle your sex drive can improve your relationship both in and out of bed. (See "Simple Ways to Spice Up Your Love Life.")

Simple Ways to Spice Up Your Love Life

- Make a date with your partner.
- Share a bath or shower.
- Give one another a massage.
- Try new lingerie or other sexy clothing.
- Buy the CD of "your song."
- Make eye contact.
- Have an honest conversation about what you like most in bed.
- Fantasize about your partner during the day.

Not in the mood   Getting "in the mood" is your responsibility. Don't expect to be ready for sex if you haven't given it a thought all day. For most women sex is as mental as it is physical, and they need to be thinking ahead and preparing for a pleasurable experience.

Lack of personal connection   No doubt about it, feeling an emotional and spiritual connection with your partner takes some work. A woman typically needs this type of connection to have a healthy, long-term sex drive. Partners need to continuously work on getting closer and staying in touch. If you have little one-on-one time with your partner, or if your partner is unfaithful or distant, you will feel a big gap in the connection, which will most likely take a toll in the intimacy department. Your commitment to resurrecting your libido must include reconnecting with your partner emotionally.

Poor body image   Few things are more damaging to a woman's sex drive than a poor self-image. If you struggle in this area, you owe it to yourself and your partner to do something about it. Begin positive self-talk and do not let negative thoughts about yourself enter your mind when you are intimate with your partner. Try telling yourself during lovemaking that you are sexual, excitable, strong, and comfortable with your body. Though it may seem simplistic, telling yourself such things will keep you moving in the right direction mentally. Remember that your brain is your most powerful sex organ. (See "Simple Exercises for Improved Body Image" on page 105.)

Sexual boredom   You must be creative. It takes time and patience to learn what your partner likes and doesn't like. Adding variety to your sex life that is pleasing, fun, and loving on both sides is invaluable to your lovemaking. (See "Simple Ways to Spice Up Your Love Life" on page 107.) Contrary to popular myth, it's not the twenty-somethings who are having all the fun. Like a fine wine, a monogamous sexual relationship can greatly improve with age. Don't discount the intimacy, trust, and skill that come with years of practice!

A Dream Date at Home

Make a date with your spouse and pull out all the stops. Use this as an opportunity to simply enjoy one another's company. This isn't the time for an in-depth "state of the union" discussion—save the conversation about any problems in the relationship for another day. This is your chance to have some one-on-one quality time with each other.

- Arrange for the kids to spend the night with friends (you can reciprocate on another weekend, to give your friends the same opportunity).

- Shop ahead of time for some sumptuous foods and something special to wear.

- Open a bottle of wine, champagne, or sparkling water or cider (use the good glasses).

- Present one another with a small, thoughtful gift.

- Share a romantic meal—nothing too heavy! (See "Foods to Fuel the Fire" on page 100.)

- Set the stage with candles and soft music in the bedroom.

- Start with a bubble bath à deux.

- Let nature take its course—relax and enjoy yourselves.

Chapter 9

The Fatigue Factor: Rejuvenate Your Thyroid

IN THIS CHAPTER:

The Powerful Thyroid

Undiagnosed, Untreated Low Thyroid Is Bad News

Low Thyroid in Perimenopause

Other Causes of Fatigue

Testing for Thyroid Disorders

Treatment Options

Carrie is a thirty-five-year-old registered nurse who works part-time and is raising three children. When she first came to my office, she voiced a common complaint: "I just don't have the energy that I once had," she sighed. Upon questioning, I learned that Carrie also had depression, dry skin, heavy periods, cold hands and feet, and poor memory and concentration. She worked at losing weight, but in the past three years had put on 20 pounds. After discussing the potential hormonal connections to her symptoms, Carrie was eager to have her levels tested.

Her hormone profile revealed that her thyroid was functioning at less than optimum output, so I started her on thyroid medication. Carrie was also educated on how to improve her thyroid function through diet, supplements, stress avoidance, and exercise. Carrie has been on thyroid replacement for two years and feels better than ever. Her skin is less dry, she has lost most of the excess weight, her thinking and memory are sharper, her periods are regular and lighter, and she has much more energy. Perhaps most important, she has come to realize that taking a pill is not a cure-all, but rather a single element in an overall commitment to total wellness through diet, exercise, hormonal balance, and stress management. Carrie also realizes that she will need to keep tabs on her thyroid for the rest of her life.

The Powerful Thyroid

Weighing in at a powerful 1 ounce, the *thyroid* is a butterfly-shaped gland at the front of the neck that extends to both sides of the Adam's apple. About the size of a walnut, it can pack the wallop of a runaway truck. Within the brain is the *hypothalamus,* which releases the signaling hormone, *TRH,* or *thyroid-releasing hormone.* This hormone travels to the *pituitary gland,* triggering the release of *TSH, or thyroid-stimulating hormone.* You got it: TSH stimulates the thyroid gland to produce hormone.

Stress, illness, and poor diet easily affect the thyroid gland, causing it to produce less thyroid hormone. When the thyroid goes into low gear, every part of the body is adversely affected. Imagine the thyroid as your engine and your metabolism its fuel, then consider what might happen if your engine grinds to minimal RPMs. You don't want to think about it. The thyroid controls the growth, temperature, and function of every cell in your body. Without thyroid hormone the body cools, slows, and, if nothing comes to its rescue, dies.

Low Thyroid Is a Common Complaint

Carrie's troubles were not unique. The well-known Colorado Thyroid Disease Prevalence Study found that as many as 13 million Americans may have undiagnosed thyroid conditions. Other studies indicate that as many as 17 percent of older American women may have the condition. Among the Colorado study's key points: An underactive thyroid—*hypothyroidism*—affects more women than men, and the risk increases with age for both. As discussed later in this chapter, low thyroid can be difficult and time-consuming to diagnose and is often missed. So-called normal ranges are broad, and women whose levels test toward the lower end have what is called *subclinical hypothyroidism.*

In his book *The Thyroid Solution,* Ridha Arem, M.D., associate professor in the Division of Endocrinology and Metabolism at Baylor College of Medicine, points out that even when test results for TSH (thyroid-stimulating hormone) fall within the normal range, hypothyroidism may exist. Dr. Arem writes that many people whose test results are dismissed as normal could continue to have symptoms of an underactive thyroid. Their moods, emotions, and overall well-being are affected by this imbalance, yet they are not receiving the care they need to get to the root of their problems. Even if the TSH level is in the lower segment of the normal range, a person may still be suffering from low-grade hypothyroidism.

Tell me about it, says Carrie and other patients whose symptoms have been dismissed. Too often the possibility that their symptoms result from low thyroid is not considered, and a simple TSH test is not even given. Instead they are prescribed antidepressants or birth control pills and are advised to eat less, exercise more, and take over-the-counter remedies for the chronic constipation that may plague them.

Medical providers must make it a point to consider a woman's symptoms along with her thyroid test results. If she has cold hands and feet, emotional disturbances, extreme fatigue, constipation, or four or five other common hypothyroidism symptoms, the possibility of low thyroid must be thoroughly investigated. The stakes of undiagnosed hypothyroidism are high.

Undiagnosed, Untreated Low Thyroid Is Bad News

An underactive thyroid can produce all kinds of unpleasant, non-life-threatening symptoms, but it also has serious long-term health implications. We know that hypothyroidism increases cholesterol, a major risk factor for heart disease. Research from the "Rotterdam Study," published in the *Annals of Internal Medicine* in 2000, indicates that older women with subclinical hypothyroidism are nearly twice as likely as women without the condition to have heart attacks and were 70 percent more likely to have hardened aortas—the body's main artery—than those with normal hormone activity.

Heart disease is not the only disturbing consequence of untreated hypo-thyroidism. According to Richard Shames, M.D., author of *Thyroid Power,* thyroid malfunction has been linked to such disorders as fibromyalgia, eczema, infertility, attention deficit disorder, phobias, loss of ambition, panic attacks, depression, and other mental illnesses.

Why Is Low Thyroid So Often Undiagnosed?

I spent several years pondering this question. It seemed obvious that low thyroid was the problem when patients consulted me with a list of symptoms pointing directly to it. Sadly, if a woman is not diagnosed early in her low-thyroid state, the problem will likely progress over the years into a significant illness that may or may not show on the blood workup, but will be putting her at risk for heart disease, osteoporosis, and other long-term complications.

Another diagnostic difficulty is that what may be normal for one woman is not normal for another. Many a patient who ends up in my office has been told that she is just depressed, stressed, overtired, or simply a low-energy person. As a result, some have settled for medication for depression, anxiety, headaches, heavy periods, and skin problems, or they have opted for surgery for menstrual difficulties. Some choose to use over-the-counter weight-loss stimulants; others perk up with caffeine and sugar. Women with severe symptoms are often popping as many as six medicines to correct problems stemming for low thyroid.

How do I know? As soon as they begin thyroid medication, they start weaning from the other drugs and eventually are freed from them.

Low Thyroid in Perimenopause

The incidence of hypothyroidism increases with age, and as many as 30 percent of women over age fifty-five may suffer from it (of course this number reflects only those who are actually diagnosed). I can't count the number of women over the past twelve years of my medical practice who have come to me with the most common complaints associated with hypothyroidism and were ultimately found to have the condition.

Perimenopausal women seem to be at an increasingly high risk for low thyroid. Though this has not been well studied, I am diagnosing more and more women in their thirties and forties with the condition. The connection between low thyroid and perimenopause could be related to stress or to the deficient diet that has become the norm for so many women. The overall hormonal changes associated with this time in life most likely have an influence, and genetics may also play a role.

Worldwide, the number one cause of hypothyroidism is low iodine in the diet. Iodine is essential for the thyroid to produce hormone, as is tyrosine, a common amino acid that is broken down from protein but can also be manufactured by the body. Because both tyrosine and iodine are in fair abundance in most American diets, the common problem of low thyroid is most likely related to our compromised immune systems.

We know that our bodies are constantly exposed to toxins through processed or contaminated foods, as well as through water and air that are tainted by our urban, industrialized environment. Exposure to continual contamination predisposes the thyroid gland to attack. Some believe that even otherwise positive exposures, such as fluoride in water to prevent tooth decay, can weaken the immune system.

Anxiety, depression, and physical, mental, and emotional overexertion can also have negative effects on the immune system, which in time can disrupt thyroid balance. Some endocrinologists suggest that viral infections are the root cause of pervasive low thyroid. Susceptibility to viral illnesses increases when our immune systems are weakened.

Stress is a major factor in the rise of hypothyroidism. Many modern women do the double shift of home and office, and our fast-paced, demanding schedules exert constant pressure and allow few mental or emotional breaks. We work harder, longer, and faster. Combine this stress overload with chemical contamination of our air, food, and water; poor exercise habits; and a fast-food, high-fat, and low-nutrient diet and what do you get? A sick, burned-out individual with chronic low energy, depression, and general malaise. One of the first hormone-producing glands to be adversely affected by toxic exposure is—you guessed it—the thyroid.

Symptoms of Low Thyroid

Every woman has distinctive metabolic needs, so the symptoms of hypo-thyroidism vary. Some women experience only vague indications such as depression or low energy. Others are afflicted with every possible symptom. Figure 9-1 on page 114 shows a checklist that I use in my office to determine if a woman is at risk for low thyroid.

If my patients notice four or more of these symptoms on a regular basis, I am suspicious of low or subclinical low thyroid. This is especially true if the symptoms are present more than three days per week.

Unfortunately, women with multiple symptoms are often labeled hypochondriacs and referred to a variety of specialists.

If you have symptoms associated with hypothyroidism, and your medical provider hasn't tested your thyroid function, ask to be tested. Numerous thyroid tests described later in this chapter can provide information essential for appropriate treatment.

Other Causes of Fatigue

Low energy is a major symptom of hypothyroidism, but it can stem from a number of conditions other than low thyroid.

Iron-deficiency anemia   This is a common cause of fatigue. If your energy is low, a simple blood test called a *CBC (complete blood count)* can quickly

Figure 9-1   Symptoms of low thyroid

Put a check next to any of the following signs that you have had consistently.

☐ Fatigue throughout the day

☐ Muscle spasms or significant muscular pain

☐ Joint pain that does not seem to be related to activity or previous injury

☐ Irritable bladder or loss of urine

☐ Swollen lymph nodes around the neck or a feeling of fullness in the throat

☐ Cold hands and feet, or general coldness

☐ Persistent depression and sadness

☐ Frequent headaches

☐ Weight gain, with no apparent change in diet or activity

☐ Inability to lose weight

☐ Impaired memory and concentration

☐ Constipation

☐ Dry, brittle hair; hair loss

☐ Dry, scaly skin

☐ Trouble conceiving a baby

☐ Hoarse voice

☐ Irregular periods—longer, heavier, more frequent

☐ No sex drive

☐ More-frequent infections that last longer

☐ Dry, gritty eyes that are sensitive to light

☐ More-frequent yawning to get oxygen

☐ Ringing in the ears (tinnitus)

☐ Recurrent sinus infections

determine whether you are anemic. Adding iron to your diet, or taking an iron supplement, can resolve the fatigue and should be started if your levels are low.

Lack of sleep   Not enough sleep or simply poor sleep are at the root of sluggishness for many women. Hectic, harried lives and an inability to relax cause some women to lie awake at night. Relaxation practices such as deep breathing, meditation, or a hot bath before bed can help, and avoiding alcohol and caffeine late in the day are important. Depression can cause sleeplessness and also result from it—one of the worst kinds of vicious circles.

Interestingly, *hyperthyroidism*—an *over*production of thyroid hormones—also causes insomnia, and low thyroid can cause sleep patterns to be intermittent and interrupted throughout the night. If insomnia is chronic and keeping you from getting seven to eight hours of sleep several nights a week, it's a good idea to talk with your medical provider. Sleep aids should not be taken on a regular basis. It is best to resolve the underlying psychological or physical problems that are preventing you from getting enough sleep.

Poor diet A poor diet can trigger fatigue in women, men, and children of all ages. By now most Americans have heard that the majority of fast foods as well as convenience and packaged foods lack the nutrients essential for good health and are instead loaded with sodium, sugar, and unhealthy fats. We have a tendency to grab sugar-laden carbohydrates that provide a quick shot of glucose, but these foods result ultimately in an energy crisis. Complex carbohydrates such as those in whole grains and fruits convert to glucose slowly in the body and provide energy over a period of hours. Simple carbohydrates, such as those in snack cakes and sugar cookies, give a spike of short-lived energy quickly followed by a crash. (See chapter 5 for more about diet.)

Lack of exercise The sedentary lifestyle is an all-too-common cause of fatigue. It may be difficult to grasp how something that uses energy also creates it, but that is exactly what regular exercise does. Exercise increases circulation, bringing increased blood flow to all the tissues and organs of the body. It is also the best way to clear your head and work through mental and emotional stress. If you want to reverse fatigue and your medical provider has told you that there are no physical reasons for your chronic tiredness, increase your activity level. Regular exercise turns fatigue into energy.

Depression This is yet another reason for low energy. Emotional difficulties can cause a tremendous amount of lethargy. Women suffering from depression have a difficult time getting out of bed in the morning and often feel worn out by midafternoon. Depression and low thyroid seem to be closely related, and when a woman reports that she is depressed, I always take a closer look at her thyroid function.

Testing for Thyroid Disorders

TSH test   The test for thyroid-stimulating hormone is an indirect way of testing the thyroid. Imagine the way a thermostat works, and you will understand TSH testing. If your thyroid does not produce enough thyroid hormone, the master pituitary gland receives the message that the pituitary needs to send a louder signal to the thyroid. So the TSH level in the blood elevates to get some action going in the thyroid. When your medical provider orders a TSH level, it can show how loud or high the signal is.

The problem is that TSH is but one piece of the diagnostic puzzle and should *not* be the only diagnostic test if hypothyroidism is a possible explanation for symptoms. This test has a ridiculously broad normal range of 0.4 to 5.6, which can vary according to the lab used. If you are having hypothyroid symptoms but test results fall in this normal range, you are considered in fine health. Many experts say that once the TSH rises above 2.5, the possibility of low thyroid should be further investigated; and if it rises above 3.0, hypothyroidism should definitely be considered. Most medical providers are not yet diagnosing this way.

I believe we need to pay attention to the TSH levels that increase above the 2.5 range. It is also interesting to note that even though the normal range is all the way up to 5.6, labs are now printing on the lab results that TSH levels above 3.0 are often associated with hypothyroidism (even though the high of normal clearly states 5.6). Fortunately, the standard normal ranges for TSH have been recently lowered, which will now allow more women to be appropriately diagnosed. There is still suspicion among thyroid specialists that a TSH above 2.0 is questionable for low thyroid.

Free T3 and free T4 hormone test   There are two thyroid hormones available in our bodies, T3 and T4. *Triiodothyronine*, also known as *T3*, is short acting and is the more potent of the two. It is T3 that controls energy in the body. *Levothyroxine*, also known as *T4*, is carried in the circulation bound to protein. It is slow acting and referred to as the storage hormone. The levels of T3 and T4 can be measured in the blood and should be ordered with the TSH. The "free T3 and T4" levels are "free" in the blood, meaning they are unbound to protein and allowed to enter target cells. Although these tests appear sensitive and are helpful when ordered with a TSH, they still may not reveal hypothyroidism.

Total T3 test   A total T3 is a more direct approach to looking into the availability of the total circulating T3 in the bloodstream. This test should be part of the thyroid workup.

Obtaining an Accurate Diagnosis

Why isn't there a uniform standard for testing thyroid hormone? I wish it were that easy, but because no two women are identical, medical providers must use several avenues to reach the correct diagnosis. I recommend a total panel of the following tests for thyroid evaluation:

- TSH (thyroid-stimulating hormone)

- Free T4

- Free T3

- Total T3

- Possibly a TRH, if necessary

TRH test   The test for thyroid-releasing hormone is expensive, but it is extremely sensitive and can detect mild or borderline hypothyroidism, often when other tests may show normal levels.

Additional Measures   Less often, advanced testing such as thyroid ultrasound and tests for thyroid antibodies may be necessary to pick up on other potential problems with the thyroid.

The following additional measures and assessments should also be carried out to complete the picture of potential low-thyroid function:

▶ Complete the symptom checklist in figure 9-1 and show it to your medical provider.

▶ Take your temperature five mornings in a row. This must be done when you first wake in the morning and before you get out of bed. Because your thyroid controls metabolism, temperature testing can provide a better picture of your body's ability to burn calories. If you are menstruating, wait until immediately after your period has ended. Place a mercury or digital thermometer in the middle of your armpit, then allow the arm to relax down over the thermometer for five minutes. Your average temperature should be at 98°F (36.7°C). If your temperature is consistently 97°F (36.1°C) or below, sluggish thyroid function could be the cause.

▶ Conduct an evaluation of your family health history in light of your current symptoms and physical signs; recognizing genetic traits can often provide a greater understanding.

Treatment Options

Several prescription medications are available for treating hypothyroidism. When starting thyroid replacement, however, realize that you will likely remain on it indefinitely. Once your levels have been stabilized, you should be evaluated at least once a year. Prescription treatment options for low thyroid include the following.

T4-only treatment   This includes commercial versions of T4 hormone:

▶ Synthroid

▶ Levothryoxine (generic)

▶ Levoxyl

▶ Unithroid

T4 can also be provided by a compounding pharmacy so that an exact dose can be formulated for you. T4 alone will usually convert to T3 in the body, so many women can use T4 tablets or capsules alone. The dose of T4 is typically 1 mcg per pound of weight, starting at one quarter of this dose and working up to the correct dose.

What About Osteoporosis?

Often when women on thyroid medicine are finally feeling better, the medical provider will note that the levels are showing that she may be getting too much and will be at risk for *osteoporosis*, or lowered bone density. If a medical provider tells you this and your levels are on the high end, you may want to learn more about the alleged osteoporosis risk.

Several years ago research data suggested that thyroid hormone replacement was associated with lowered bone density. As a result, most providers became wary of the medicine and began seriously undertreating hypothyroidism. Recent research using more-sophisticated testing shows no correlation between thyroid hormone medicine and osteoporosis, even at higher doses. The irony is that for years women have been radically underdiagnosed and undertreated based in part on outdated research. There is some concern that untreated low thyroid may actually be a *cause* of osteoporosis, which is the very opposite of what medical providers have thought for years.

T3 and T4 combination Slower-acting T4 and faster-acting T3 can be combined into a capsule and formulated according to prescription at a compounding or conventional pharmacy. The advantage of using a compounding pharmacy is that doses of either hormone can be adjusted according to individual needs and be prepared for sustained release. Armour, Naturthroid, and Westroid are brand names of prescription medications that combine T3 and T4 in a fixed ratio, which may not be ideal for many women.

T3-only treatment It is possible to use just T3 for treatment of low thyroid. Some women have a T3 deficiency and not a T4, which is another reason for having the full thyroid panel. Cytomel, which is a commercial tablet of T3, is available in only two strengths. It is an immediate-release formula, which necessitates dosing several times per day. A more flexible approach is have the T3 formulated by a pharmacy to a personalized strength in a sustained-release capsule. This is often the medication of choice when a T3 deficiency is noted. It has a potent, fast-acting effect that is also being used to treat women suffering from chronic fatigue, fibromyalgia, and depression.

Typically, the body converts T4 into T3, although in some people this conversion does not take place adequately. The 5'-deiodinase enzyme that is necessary for the conversion of T4 to T3 may be reduced in someone who has a deficiency in selenium, iron, boron, or zinc or even in women who lead stressful lives, often producing too much cortisol.

Over-the-counter options:

▶ Thyroid Glandular (desiccated thyroid with active ingredients removed)

▶ Thyroid 130

▶ GF Thyroid

▶ Thyroplex

Homeopathic remedies:

▶ Thyroid 6x (pellets)

▶ Thyroid R-6 (liquid)

A trained compounding pharmacist is able to create a bioidentical, natural thyroid combination best suited to your needs, and the dosing can be altered as necessary. Such a compound does not use pork or beef thyroid by-products.

Which Treatment Is Most Effective?

As you can see, there is no perfect combination of medicine that is effective in every case. It will take some time to get the levels correct, and a change in medication may be in order if side effects are present or if the low-thyroid symptoms are not arrested. Keep in mind that juggling brands, medication types, and dosing amounts may be necessary until the symptoms are relieved. Your healthcare provider should work with you to get you there safely.

Natural Supplements for Hypothyroidism

Women who have mild hypothyroidism, or who have low-thyroid symptoms without a confirming diagnosis, can use the following supplements:

Vitamin A   10,000 to 20,000 IU per day

Vitamin C   500 to 2,000 mg per day

B-complex   100 mg complex; capsules or sublingual drops (see "Vitamin and Herbal Supplements" in appendix B for purchasing options)

Flaxseed   4,000 to 6,000 mg per day of flaxseed oil capsules; 1 tablespoon per day of flaxseed oil; or 2 to 3 tablespoons per day of ground flaxseed

Chromium picolinate   200 to 800 mcg per day

Zinc   25 to 50 mg per day

Selenium   100 to 200 mcg per day

Copper   1 mg per day

Natural vitamin E (d-alpha tocopherol)   400 IU per day

Tyrosine   1,000 mg per day

Kelp   500 mg tablet containing 225 mcg iodine (avoid this if you have autoimmune thyroiditis)

An additional option is natural thyroid glandular extract or stimulating supplements (see appendix B for purchasing options). Always use a 100 percent natural extract.

The Quick-Fix Plan for Energy

- Sleep seven to nine hours every night. Try to go to bed and get up at the same times every night and morning.

- Eat breakfast every morning, with at least 14 to 21 grams of protein plus a good low-sugar carbohydrate that is rich in fiber. Sprouted grain toast and oatmeal are good choices.

- Eliminate sugar and caffeine because they stress and weaken the immune system, causing even less support to the thyroid.

- Eat small frequent meals.

- Quit smoking.

- Limit alcohol to one or two drinks per week.

- Identify one daily strategy to manage stress.

- Breathe, breathe, breathe—your thyroid needs oxygenation to work well.

- Eat thyroid-promoting foods: Include adequate protein, yogurt, wheat germ, whole grains (sprouted wheat instead of flour), nuts, seeds, dark greens, brewer's yeast, seaweed, and wheat germ oil.

Medicine alone will rarely make you well. Emotional, spiritual, and physical health are inseparable. If you continue with unhealthful eating habits, refuse to exercise, and are assaulted by unrelieved stress, your chances for optimal health are greatly compromised. But by eating healthier, exercising, and minimizing stress, you'll look younger, feel better, and most likely be happier as well.

Other Hazards of Perimenopause

IN THIS CHAPTER:

Surviving Hot Flashes and Night Sweats

What Can I Do About Irregular Periods?

Hope for Thinning Hair and Hair Loss

Banishing Breast Tenderness

The Cure for Vaginal Dryness and Irritation

Treating Migraines and Other Headaches

Bladder Control 101

Getting a Good Night's Sleep

Imagine the embarrassment of giving a presentation or lecture in front of a roomful of people when, all of a sudden, your body temperature spikes, your face lights up like a firecracker, and you break out in sweat. Such hot flashes are fairly common among perimenopausal women and have caused more than one woman to flee the room.

Night sweats can be annoying and disturbing, too. The disruption of sleep patterns wreaks havoc with your body and sets in motion a domino effect: Sleep deprivation can cause loss of memory and concentration, then fatigue, irritability, and sometimes depression. Fatigue can lead to poor eating habits; it is way easier to reach for a pastry for breakfast than to prepare oatmeal. Stress increases as women worry about not getting a good night's sleep. Often women in perimenopause can go weeks without a night sweat, but then they start up again.

Surviving Hot Flashes and Night Sweats

The ebb and flow of female hormones during perimenopause are responsible for hot flashes and night sweats. Most women I work with experience these symptoms at two different times each month. The first time occurs during ovulation, when the estrogen level rises, then falls. The second time can occur a few days before a woman gets her period, but sometimes can last the full two weeks leading up to it. At both times hormone levels—especially progesterone—are on the decline. When progesterone is not in balance with estrogen, hot flashes and night sweats can cause the hallmark "power surges" of perimenopause.

A basic difference between a woman in perimenopause and a woman in her twenties is that the perimenopausal woman often has lowered levels of progesterone—and sometimes estrogen—at specific points in her cycle.

When a woman begins having hot flashes, it's a sure sign that her hormone levels are out of sync. Having hormone levels tested is the first plan of action in banishing these annoying symptoms. A simple blood test helps identify whether progesterone or estrogen levels are low before your period or if your estrogen levels are high during ovulation. Once your levels have been tested, you can decide to treat symptoms either with supplements or, more aggressively, with natural hormones. Your decision should be based on the following considerations.

Factors Under Your Control

First, your lifestyle may be contributing to hot flashes and night sweats. Alcohol consumption, too much stress, too little exercise, even setting the room temperature too high—all can contribute to hot flashes and night sweats.

Alcohol consumption   Alcohol can disturb sleep patterns and significantly alter blood-sugar levels, especially when consumed late in the evening. Even without perimenopausal hormone fluctuations, alcohol can cause hot flashes and night sweats. If you like a nightcap in the evening, try having just one drink, and be sure to eat something with it. A little food (especially protein) helps balance your blood sugar and keep insulin levels lower, to dull the alcohol's effect. But be sure your snack is not a high-sugar, high-carbohydrate item. A handful of almonds or a slice of reduced-fat cheese with a whole-wheat cracker can help balance the effects of the sugar in the alcohol.

Stress This is probably the leading cause of hot flashes and night sweats. As explained in chapter 6, our bodies react to persistently high stress levels by releasing cortisol into the bloodstream. Unfortunately, when cortisol is released continuously, it alters the female hormonal balance, causing erratic and inconsistent estrogen levels which in turn cause hot flashes and night sweats. Women often feel more stressed just before their periods; and when their ability to cope with stress is altered, that out-of-control feeling takes over. And when you feel out of control, you get even more stressed, which leads to a heightened feeling of being out of control, which leads to . . . well, you get the picture.

Doctors often find that stress is the primary cause behind many problems women face during perimenopause. But, as discussed in chapter 6, stress *can* be managed. Taking time for yourself—with a long bath, a 20-minute walk, some deep breathing, or a fun activity—is a very effective stress reliever. It's amazing what happens when you take just ten minutes to relax and breathe deeply. Getting oxygen to your brain, after unconsciously holding your breath all day due to stress, can save you from going over the edge. Balancing work, pleasure, family, and home is part of balancing your body's chemistry. Don't expect your hormones to get into balance if you aren't!

Environment To further handle hot flashes and night sweats, try setting your thermostat to a cooler temperature. Studies show that people rest best at night when a room is set at 68°F (20°C). Use minimal covers, keeping your body warm but your head and feet cool. Even a slight change in temperature can trigger night sweats, so start cool; then, when your body warms up, you are less apt to wake up in a sweat.

Exercise Daily exercise is an excellent stress reducer. Exercise releases endorphins that help you feel tranquil and contribute to a sense of well-being. Women who consistently exercise appear to suffer fewer symptoms from hormonal imbalance.

Supplements for Regulating Hot Flashes and Night Sweats

Consider taking one or a combination of the following supplements, which have been found to regulate hot flashes and night sweats.

Black cohosh Although this herb doesn't restore estrogen balance, it can help reduce hot flashes and night sweats.

Evening primrose oil or flaxseed oil   These oils, available in capsule form, can moisturize your skin, help your brain function, and reduce cravings. They can also help regulate sweats and hot flashes during the day.

Calcium-magnesium   Available in both capsule and liquid form, a good dose of calcium-magnesium taken before bedtime promotes healthy sleep. I prefer the liquid form because it doesn't bother the stomach and works well to relax the body and enhance sleep.

Vitamin E   Taken daily, 400 to 800 IU of vitamin E can help eliminate hot flashes and get you through the night without sweating. It works especially well when combined with calcium-magnesium and flaxseed oil.

Red clover   This supplement contains weak estrogen compounds that are often enough to improve estrogen levels.

Soy supplements   Extremely popular in Asia, soy supplements have been shown to reduce night sweats and hot flashes. The suggested form to take is isoflavones, at 50 to 150 mg daily. Although not effective for all women, soy works well for some. Give it two weeks, then decide if it's worth continuing.

Estrogen or progesterone   A prescription of progesterone or estradiol (or combined estrogens such as bi-est and tri-est) in a bioidentical form that's been formulated by a compounding pharmacy can eliminate hot flashes and night sweats entirely. These prescriptions can be used in small amounts right before the period, when hot flashes and night sweats are most likely at their worst. They can also be used in small doses throughout the cycle. It is very important to start with a small amount and increase when needed as instructed by your physician. The sublingual drop form and the topical cream or gel allow you to alter your dose as needed. When hot flashes or night sweats are under control, you can ask your medical provider to reduce the dosage.

Estrogen patch   When symptoms mostly occur the week before the period, the patch, available by prescription, can be put on and left for the entire week before your period begins. Patches are available in a variety of strengths to match whatever dose is needed to control symptoms.

Check out your medicine cabinet. If you get hot flashes throughout your menstrual cycle and don't think you are experiencing the hormonal changes of perimenopause, one of your medications could be the culprit. Some medicines, such as vasodilators, calcium channel blockers, certain high-blood-pressure medications, fertility drugs, and breast cancer medications, can cause flushing and sweating.

What Can I Do About Irregular Periods?

If all other problems have been ruled out, and your doctor believes that your periods are irregular due to perimenopause, there are still steps you can take.

As discussed in chapter 2, too much estrogen and a deficiency of progesterone can cause irregular periods or heavy bleeding. A full monthly menstrual cycle—from the beginning of one period to the beginning of the next—can range from twenty-one to forty-two days. By the time women are in their forties, those who have had twenty-eight-day cycles notice that their periods either come closer together or get farther apart. Examples of irregular bleeding that can occur during perimenopause include:

▶ Bleeding or spotting midway between periods

▶ Bleeding or spotting two or three days before or after the period

▶ Bleeding only every three months or skipping periods

▶ Bleeding every fourteen to twenty-one days

▶ Experiencing heavy periods that leave you feeling worn out, or having heavier and more painful periods than in the past

If your periods are irregular, I suggest getting a hormonal blood test eighteen to twenty-one days after the first day of the previous period. This test should indicate whether your estrogen level is too high or your progesterone level is too low. For instance, if the test is drawn at least five to seven days before your next period is expected to start, and the estradiol level is above 240 pg/ml, your estrogen level is too high. If your progesterone level is below 5 pg/ml, it is too low and most likely is causing your irregular bleeding. (See chapter 3 for more information about test results.)

Natural progesterone, prescribed by your healthcare practitioner, is the best treatment for irregular bleeding. Treatment often begins twelve to fourteen days after the first day of your last period. Progesterone can be taken until your next period begins, or until day 28 to day 30 of your cycle. With the help of your medical provider, you should manipulate the dose and timing until the problem is under control.

Some medical providers prescribe lower doses of birth control pills to reinitiate periods or to stop breakthrough bleeding. Although this works for some, other women may feel worse using the synthetic hormones found in most birth control pills. Getting to the bottom of the problem by testing hormone levels and then balancing the hormones through treatment and lifestyle changes is the best approach.

Some women with irregular bleeding may prefer options besides progesterone. In such cases, the following alternatives can be used instead of or as supplements to progesterone.

Fiber Fiber binds with excessive levels of estrogen and helps the digestive tract eliminate excess estrogen. Increasing fiber also improves bowel function.

Supplements There are various supplements available that improve the health and function of your liver (the organ that metabolizes and excretes hormones). These include:

▶ Alpha lipoic acid (a powerful antioxidant)

▶ Milk thistle

▶ Amino acids methionine and cysteine

▶ Flaxseed oil supplements

▶ Licorice root

▶ Shepherd's purse (a natural supplement for heavy bleeding)

DIM Di-indolylmethane (DIM) and indole-3-carbinol (I3C) have been shown in clinical tests to reduce excessive levels of estrogen and to possibly reduce the transformation of estrogen into precancerous metabolites.

Stress reduction Again, stress can cause irregular periods. Reducing or at least managing it is an important step in overall health.

Exercise Increase your amount of daily exercise. Also consider weight-resistance training to build muscle mass and improve metabolism.

Hope for Thinning Hair and Hair Loss

Losing hair is a significant problem for some perimenopausal women, but there are many reasons why hair falls out or becomes dry and thin. The good news is you can treat your tresses and help prevent future hair loss.

Hair 101

Our scalps are covered with hair follicles that produce tiny hairs, which take up to two months to grow an inch. Hormones can affect the health of hair follicles, and estrogen is the key to growing long hair. During perimenopause, lowering levels of estrogen can cause the thinning of head hair. Although it's normal to lose about a hundred hair follicles from the scalp each day, fortunately, our scalps contain 1 million of them.

Some experts who treat patients with *alopecia* (early hair loss) suggest the "pencil" test to evaluate the true loss of head hair. When you part your hair, if the space is as wide as a pencil, early hair loss may be a concern. If your part is thin and not showing signs of significant widening, it's likely your hair loss is normal. Another way to determine hair loss is to notice how thick your ponytail is (assuming you have one, of course). If your ponytail is half the diameter it used to be, early hair loss could be occurring.

Your doctor must determine the cause of hair loss before he or she can develop a treatment plan that works. A hormonal analysis will determine if hormone levels are in balance and not the cause of the underlying problem. When women have sudden drops in estrogen, or an excess of other female hormones such as testosterone, head hair can be significantly affected. Ask your doctor to check levels of thyroid, testosterone, estradiol, DHEA-S (sulfate), progesterone, and androstendione to rule out hormonal causes of hair loss or thinning. If your hormone levels are within normal ranges, the following suggestions can help slow hair loss and begin a regrowth cycle.

Diet, Exercise, and Stress Reduction

Improve diet Follow the dietary plan in chapter 5 to help balance blood-sugar levels, reduce insulin, and improve the health of your skin and hair cells. Elevated insulin levels, known as *insulin resistance,* are a known cause of hair loss. Improving your diet is paramount because food is a drug that will either work for you or against you.

Reduce body fat   Excessive body fat can cause higher androgen levels, which are related to hair loss. Getting your body fat below 28 percent will reduce androgen and insulin production and result in less hair thinning and loss. Reducing body fat with also make your energy level soar. (See chapter 5 for more on weight, fat loss, and exercise.)

Manage stress   Stress is the most common external cause of hair loss. Review chapter 6 and make an effort to manage your stress with practices that routinely put you into a calm state. (See specifically "The Quick-Fix Plan for Stress" in chapter 6.)

Supplements

The following supplements have been found to help slow hair loss and thinning and are worth a try.

Saw palmetto   This tropical berry helps block the conversion of testosterone to DHT, which is believed to cause hair loss when testosterone levels are high or when the hair follicle has increased sensitivity to testosterone.

Biotin   Although no studies have documented its effectiveness for hair growth, biotin has been hailed as a supplement that can improve the health of hair follicles.

B-complex   The combination of B vitamins seems to improve hair health and may prevent overall hair loss by preventing breakage and splitting.

Prescription Medications

The following prescription medications have been shown to combat hair loss.

Spironolactone   This medication can be taken orally or used topically. The oral medication, also known as Aldactone, reduces blood levels of testosterone and could prevent hair loss or possibly promote regrowth. The topical version of Spironolactone, which is more appropriate for reducing androgen activity at the skin cell site (the hair follicle), can prevent hair loss and promote regrowth.

Topical steroids   Using steroids such as Kenolog spray (triamcinolone) on the scalp can suppress the production of androgens and increase the number of head hairs. Applying steroids to the scalp can arrest hair loss over time. Within ninety days, new growth should appear.

Birth control pills   Taking the pill can reduce free levels of testosterone, thereby reducing hair loss caused by androgens. Taking the pill primarily to reduce hair loss is not recommended, however.

Progesterone   Taking progesterone can help restore the body's estrogen and progesterone balance and thus create a healthier environment for the hair follicle. Progesterone also contributes to the health of the sebaceous gland, which is attached to the hair follicle.

Estrogen   Gradual or sudden estrogen loss, whether following the birth of a baby or during perimenopause, can lead to hair loss. The loss of estrogen often is associated with a rise in testosterone, which can further promote hair loss. Using small amounts of estrogen replacement therapy can increase the growth of estrogen and help stop hair loss.

Rogaine   This and or other hair-loss prescriptions must be taken for at least four months before results of hair regrowth are evident. These products can be applied as a spray and can be used in a generic form, which is less expensive.

Hair-care Products

Consult your hairdresser regarding products that improve the health and vitality of hair follicles and restore luster to the hair shaft.

Banishing Breast Tenderness

Women's breasts are loaded with hormonal receptors that are affected by even small changes in hormonal balance. The breast's anatomy, which can be a mystery to women who detect lumps and wonder about cancer, is shown in figure 10-1 on page 132. Breasts contain multiple lobes, which are divided into smaller lobules; these lobules are then divided into smaller bulbs that produce milk. The area between the lobes is filled with fat, and for some women this fat tissue is more generous. Small-breasted women may mistake the fat-filled areas between the lobes as breast lumps.

Breasts go through multiple changes each month that are influenced by hormones, and each monthly cycle causes a different effect. As a woman's period approaches, her breasts prepare for breastfeeding. Under the influence of estrogen and progesterone, tiny ducts close to the nipple fill with fluid, which

Figure 10-1   Anatomy of the breast

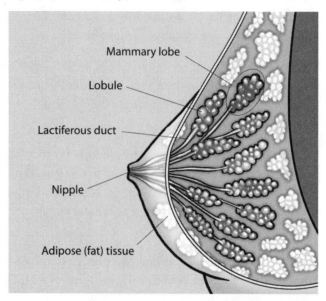

Mammary lobe

Lobule

Lactiferous duct

Nipple

Adipose (fat) tissue

causes swelling and a feeling of fullness. It can also cause breast tenderness, which often diminishes once the period has started. The breasts can also be filled with tiny cysts that collect fluid and cause lumpiness. These cysts can make the breasts sore most of the time, but particularly so just before the period.

If you experience sore or lumpy breasts, have a doctor check for possible medical problems. Once your doctor determines that your breast tenderness is noncancerous, there are a number of things you can do to reduce soreness in the breasts or nipple areas each month.

Change your diet   Four simple steps can make a difference in the degree of breast pain you experience:

▶ Reduce your fat intake—especially saturated fats and animal fats. Limit your total dietary fat to no more than 25 to 30 percent.

▶ Eliminate caffeine. This will reduce fibrocystic breast pain. Caffeine includes coffee, tea, chocolate, soft drinks, and certain medications.

▶ Cut back on animal meat, unless it's hormone-free.

▶ Reduce your consumption of processed or "prepared" foods that are high in sodium and other ingredients that the body can't use.

Take vitamin E   Try a supplement of 400 to 800 IU daily for the two weeks leading up to your period. Vitamin E has been shown to reduce breast pain associated with cyclical changes.

Try essential fatty acids   These supplements include evening primrose oil, omega-3 fatty acids, and flaxseed oil capsules. Take 1,000 to 3,000 mg daily or for the two weeks leading up to the period.

Keep exercising   Studies show that women who consistently exercise have fewer breast problems and lower incidence of breast cancer.

Reduce body fat   Estrogen is stored in fat cells. When women have a high body-fat percentage, estrogen production can be enhanced, causing more breast tenderness.

Get tested   Have your hormones tested for possible high estradiol and low progesterone.

The Cure for Vaginal Dryness and Irritation

There is no reason why any woman should endure the unpleasant effects of vaginal dryness and irritation to the external female genitalia. Vaginal dryness in perimenopausal woman can have many causes, including medications such as antidepressants, excessive caffeine, decongestants, oral contraceptives, stress, lack of foreplay, and specific hormonal deficiencies, such as of estradiol and testosterone.

First, to rule out other possible causes of irritation or pain, such as an infection or a lesion, it's important that your doctor diagnose the problem as "vaginal atrophy," "atrophic changes," or estrogen deficiency. Once a diagnosis of atrophy or thinning of the tissues is made, it is fairly easy to remedy the problem. Treating vaginal/vulvar atrophy will also help with bladder control, lubrication, and prevention of vaginal infections (such as yeast and bacteria overgrowth).

By improving tissue health and increasing the area's elasticity, moistness, and padding, you will again be able to enjoy sex, which will no longer be painful. More natural lubrication also leads to improved sensation.

Hormone Treatments

The genital area contains multiple estrogen and testosterone receptors that depend on adequate levels of these hormones to keep them healthy, plump, and youthful. Estrogen and testosterone promote adequate blood flow in the pelvic organs and surrounding tissues, they help maintain a healthy pH balance in the vaginal area, and they keep healthy bacteria in check and working to your benefit. If your blood levels of estrogen are normal, your tissues can still benefit from the use of estriol, a weak natural form of estrogen.

Using estriol vaginal cream formulated by a compounding pharmacy is the best treatment for vaginal dryness. This product is not available through large pharmaceutical companies, so it must be specially formulated by a pharmacy that is skilled at compounding (see "Compounding Pharmacies" in appendix A). Estriol can be applied to the vagina internally with an applicator or used on the external tissues for improved elasticity, especially at the vaginal opening. Most of my patients use it both internally and externally because it has a powerful effect on the mucous membranes. If the cream or gel is applied externally, it promotes a healthier, more lubricated and pliable vagina.

Women typically use estriol cream nightly for two to three weeks, then once or twice a week thereafter. Some women need to use it more regularly, whereas others find that once or twice a month is enough to maintain adequate moisture and prevent vaginal thinning. Unlike estradiol creams—the traditional hormone therapy—estriol won't build up the uterine lining. Therefore, you don't have to combine it with progesterone to protect yourself against uterine cancer.

For women who struggle with vaginal dryness and loss of sexual sensation, or for those who experience extreme dryness and irritation, adding testosterone to the estriol cream helps. Applying just testosterone externally in gel form can also improve tissue tone and lubrication.

Women who prefer not to use either hormone can rub vitamin E oil daily into external tissues to improve their health. Other vaginal moisturizers, such as Replens, Astro-glide, and K-Y Jelly, are available over-the-counter.

Something as simple as relaxing and going a little slower during sex can further enhance vaginal and vulvar lubrication. Natural lubrication usually takes a little longer at first, so you and your partner should take time to enjoy each other sexually. Start with a relaxing massage that leads to foreplay. Let your glands moisturize the vaginal area before you jump into the act.

Treating Migraines and Other Headaches

The topic of headaches alone could fill an entire book. The headaches I address here are the cyclical kind—those that occur in some sort of pattern. They usually happen before the period or around ovulation. Often these cyclic headaches are related to hormones. When I treat women who complain of significant headaches—whether they are migraines or tension headaches—their relief is significant when their hormones are finally balanced.

Headaches that are hormonally based are often associated with plummeting estrogen levels. These dropoffs most often occur before the period and at ovulation. Low levels of progesterone can also be the culprit. To make matters more confusing, estrogen dominance, which occurs when estrogen levels are overpowering progesterone levels, can also cause headaches. Some specialists believe that low levels of *serotonin*, the "feel-good" brain chemical, are associated with increased complaints of headaches. Interestingly, estrogen helps regulate serotonin levels in the blood. So it is very possible that with poor estrogen regulation, serotonin also may be low, therefore inducing headaches. This most likely is the reason why more than two-thirds of migraine sufferers in the United States are women and why women are cyclically prone to migraines.

Because there are different types of headaches, it is best to have them formally diagnosed as either migraine- or tension-based. Migraine headaches cause severe, pounding pain that can change your vision and cause sensitivity to light and sound. Often they leave you feeling sick to your stomach and unable to move. A tension headache most often feels as if there is a clamp around your head that is tightened to such an extreme that it causes tension, pressure, and pain.

Hormone-related headaches   If you suspect that your headaches are hormone-related, have your estrogen and progesterone levels tested between five and seven days before your period is to begin. Having a doctor run a thyroid panel helps ensure that thyroid troubles are not at the root of your problem. Once your test levels are evaluated, your doctor may suggest taking a small dose of estrogen at ovulation or just before your period.

The dose could be in the form of tri-estrogen drops, an estrogen patch, or even an estrogen cream or capsule. Start with a dose of 0.625 to 1.25 mg of tri-estrogen or bi-estrogen (compounded natural estrogen) once or twice daily for five to seven days before your period. You may also need to take a dose for two to three days at ovulation (around day 14 of the cycle). If estradiol levels in the blood are below 70 pg/ml before your period—or if you're not having periods and two different samples show a level of less than 70 pg/ml—these forms of estrogen could be used as a trial.

Another option is to take progesterone in a capsule, as a cream, or as sublingual drops. Progesterone can be taken with or without the estrogen.

If blood progesterone levels are below 4 pg/ml the week before your period, progesterone replacement should be considered. Take natural, bioidentical, plant-based progesterone—not the synthetic type, which can cause unwanted side effects (including migraine headaches). Have your doctor also test levels of other hormones, such as DHEA-S and free testosterone.

Preventive Measures for Headaches

Reduce stress   Stress is another cause of headaches. Using stress reduction techniques and, of course, practicing regular deep breathing helps reduce excessive output of cortisol, the stress hormone.

Drink water   Dehydration is another common cause of headaches, and I continually urge my patients to increase their water intake. Drinking water can relieve a headache that occurs in the afternoon, when you are most apt to become dehydrated. Remember, when you begin to feel thirsty, you are already mildly dehydrated, and headaches are one side effect of dehydration.

Exercise   Regular exercise can reduce the intensity and frequency of both migraine and stress-tension headaches. *Endorphins,* those feel-good brain chemicals that are released during exercise, counterbalance the ill effects of headaches. Exercise is the best stress-buster available to humans.

Eat regularly   Eating regularly can eliminate the throbbing headaches caused by low blood sugar. The blood sugar/glucose level in the blood is best kept at an equilibrium throughout the day. Try to eat a small meal four or five times a day, and avoid sugar and excessively starchy foods. When you include protein, eat more fruits and veggies, and substitute whole-wheat for white bread, you'll have more energy, less fatigue, and fewer headaches. In fact, I have helped patients completely eliminate headaches with this lifestyle change alone.

Additional measures   Other measures that aid in the relief and deterrence of headaches include but are not limited to acupuncture, biofeedback, and essential fatty acids. Herbal treatments such as feverfew and magnesium, and herbal teas such as chamomile, ginger, and valerian root, can also help. Your doctor can discuss with you the many migraine headache medications now available. Other causes of headaches will and should be ruled out by your medical provider before attempting any of these treatments.

Bladder Control 101

As you reach the perimenopausal years, your estrogen level begins to decline and you will notice less bladder control. Even in their thirties, many women notice a lack of control, and it appears to be a growing problem with women today. The reasons why women lose their urine more easily, or experience frequency of urination, are not completely understood. What we do know, however, is that when hormones begin to change, the bladder's elasticity, tissue health, and sphincter control are significantly affected.

Apply hormone cream   Multiple estrogen receptors are hidden in the walls of the bladder, the urethra (the tube leading out of the bladder), and the meatus (the external area where urine comes out). When estrogen levels begin to fall or fluctuate, bladder control can be affected because these tissues are dependent on estrogen.

Regularly applying estriol (bioidentical compounded estrogen) in a cream form to external tissues can help prevent the loss of estrogen and improve bladder control. There is growing evidence that applying testosterone gel to the external areas can additionally help with bladder control and improve circulation to the tissues.

Drink water and eliminate caffeine   Other helpful measures include increasing water intake to help dilute the urine: The more concentrated the urine, the more it will irritate the bladder. So drink up. Eliminating caffeine, whether it's in the form of coffee, tea, cola, carbonated beverages, chocolate, or a medication that contains caffeine, will help too. Caffeine in the system can cause the bladder to spasm, causing urine leakage. It's like holding a teacup filled with tea while shaking your hand. It's only a matter of time before you spill the tea.

Establish a better-bladder-control program   If you are urinating every one to two hours, try to wait longer—up to five to ten minutes longer each week—between urinations. If done properly, this retraining will help you gain more bladder control and produce greater elasticity. If you are not able to wait one minute longer after you feel the initial sensation to urinate, consider seeing a urologist for an evaluation of a nerve problem.

Do Kegel exercises   Consider doing pelvic muscle exercises. There are different methods, but I suggest starting with this simple practice: Every time you start to urinate, stop the urine flow and try to hold it for a few seconds. The bladder muscles that help you stop urination are the same ones you use to hold your bladder in place and control urination.

Another way to perform these exercises is to tighten the muscles that help close the vaginal, anal, and urethral areas. Perform these exercises three times daily: Tighten for ten seconds, release, then repeat nine more times. Consider purchasing a device known as the Kegel Master, which you place in your vagina and adjust to the tension you can master at that time. Over time, increase the tension as your muscles become stronger. You can also consider the Myself system, a pelvic muscle trainer (PMT) for women with bladder control problems. It teaches and motivates women to effectively perform pelvic muscle exercises (commonly known as Kegels) to strengthen the muscles that control urination. Formerly available by prescription, Myself is now the first FDA-cleared over-the-counter solution for bladder control. (See "Products for Incontinence" in appendix C.)

Additional measures   Other methods to increase bladder control include biofeedback, magnetic stimulation, bladder-control medications, incontinence rings, and pessaries (diaphragm-like devices inserted into the vagina to hold the bladder in place). Again, an appropriate diagnosis by your gynecological or urological healthcare provider should identify the problem prior to treatment.

Getting a Good Night's Sleep

Sleepless nights eventually leave you irritable, overweight, depressed, chronically fatigued, mentally dulled, hormonally imbalanced, and lacking motivation. Not a pretty picture. More Americans are suffering from insomnia and sleepless nights than ever before. It's not too hard to imagine why. Stress, excessive caffeine, a sedentary lifestyle, and a poor diet that lacks most of the essential vitamins and nutrients needed to stabilize our hormone output—all cause sleep deprivation.

Why Is Sleep So Important?

Our bodies handle many important tasks while we sleep. Most important is maintaining our body's *circadian rhythm.* This "body clock" regulates our sleep pattern; it tells us when we should sleep, when we should awaken, when we should have a bowel movement, and when we should be at our peak performance. It also regulates specific hormones in the body. When we get fewer

Establishing Better Sleep Patterns

Synchronize your body clock   Try to go to sleep and wake up at the same time each day to regulate your internal clock.

Increase daytime or morning exercise   Using your head all week at work and dealing with stress is the bane of a good night's sleep. Balance headwork with bodywork to promote restful sleep.

Avoid caffeine   If you can't eliminate caffeine entirely, at least stop consuming it after noon.

Set the stage   Make your sleeping area very dark and cool. People sleep best at 68°F (20°C) in a dark room.

Avoid alcohol   Although it may help you feel drowsy, alcohol interrupts the depth of your sleep and will keep you awake during the night.

Try supplements   There are many supplements to help you sleep. These include the following:

- Calcium-magnesium (liquid is best) at bedtime; try 500 to 1,500 mg of calcium with at least 400 mg of magnesium

- Valerian root for calming effect; try 150 to 300 mg in a capsule form that is standardized to 0.8% valerenic acid at bedtime

- 5-HTP (50 to 150 mg at bedtime) to help increase serotonin, which also helps increase melatonin (the sleep hormone)

- Melatonin (sublingual drops), in a compounded form or over-the-counter; try a 2 mg time-release dose at around 8 p.m. or a sublingual dose of 0.5 to 3 mg at bedtime

- DHEA-S (a precursor to estrogen and testosterone), 10 to 25 mg, taken in the morning

than seven hours of sleep per night, our internal body clock becomes confused about when we should go to sleep and wake up. Sleep deprivation also causes unstable patterns of sleepiness and fatigue. The brain does not release the chemicals necessary for hormonal balance, and the body is unable to produce the necessary cortisol that helps us wake up in the morning.

Sleep-promoting hormones   Hormones necessary for promoting restful sleep include estrogen, progesterone, DHEA-S, melatonin, serotonin, and insulin. These hormone levels should be checked prior to your period. (If you are no longer having periods, obtain one or two samples at two different times of the month.) Regulating hormonal balance can help you get a good night's sleep again. Women who are perimenopausal often need progesterone to stabilize their sleep patterns. You may want to start with a prescription or an over-the-counter progesterone cream. Use progesterone cyclically, before your period, to see if your sleep patterns change.

Consider medications   Taking sleep medications for short-term insomnia can help break the pattern of sleeplessness and get you back on track, but be careful not to overuse these medications.

Regular sex   Also consider regular lovemaking—the most incredible sleeping agent. Women who engage in regular sex (three times per week on average) have more-sustained sleep patterns and less insomnia. In addition, women who enjoy a steady diet of sex have fewer wrinkles, less stress, less depression, and greater contentment (and most likely a happier home life).

The 12-Week Hormone-Balancing Plan

I n my office twelve weeks is a magical time frame. Our weight management program is a 12-week plan, incorporating a cleansing diet for the first two weeks, followed by weekly changes that ultimately result in an excellent long-term eating strategy. The hormonal overhaul plan is also set up for twelve weeks. First the patient is medically evaluated, consulted regarding her problems and concerns, tested via blood samples for hormone imbalances, then scheduled back into the office to discuss lab results.

An individualized plan is developed for each patient, and often hormones are formulated to meet unique needs. A follow-up visit and repeat labs are done within the twelve weeks. Throughout the process we work with patients to help them incorporate dietary changes, develop a game plan for stress management, and revamp their personal schedules so they are better able to care for themselves. It is amazing what can be accomplished in such a short time, and women who choose to follow one of our 12-week plans are rarely disappointed.

This book was designed to help you navigate a 12-week plan on your own or with the help of a medical provider who is in agreement with the principles discussed. Each chapter can help you put together a game plan for renewal, and this epilogue recaps the book's basic guidelines. In a short time you can feel better and gain control of your health and your life. You may choose to stick with the magic number of twelve weeks or tackle the programs for a shorter or longer time frame, depending on your current situation. The important thing to recognize is that *you must stick with it.* See "The 12-Week Hormonal Overhaul" and "The 12-Week Diet Overhaul," which recap the basic guidelines to lead you to better health and wellness.

The 12-Week Hormonal Overhaul

Identify possible hormonal imbalances   Check off the following symptoms you may be experiencing.

☐ *Estrogen dominance:* Irritability, fibroids, fibrocystic breasts, heavy periods, weight gain, acne, depression, anger, PMS

☐ *Progesterone deficiency:* PMS, irregular periods, bloating, weight gain, fatigue, breast pain, depression

☐ *Testosterone deficiency:* Fatigue, low sex drive, reduced endurance or strength, loss of muscle mass

☐ *Testosterone excess:* Rage, irritability, facial or chest hair, loss of head hair

Have your hormones tested   Testing should occur in the last half of your menstrual cycle, or about eighteen to twenty-one days after the first day of the period. Tests should include estradiol, progesterone, free testosterone, and a full thyroid panel, including a TSH, Free T4, Free T3, and Total T3. Please do not be apologetic about insisting on these tests. Each is important in discovering your underlying issues.

Discuss your test results with your medical provider   Use the normal value ranges given in figures 2-1, 2-3, and 2-5 to determine if you are in the optimal range for the hormones being analyzed.

Develop a treatment plan to correct hormonal imbalances   Obviously, this will be more difficult if your medical provider is not skilled in treating with natural hormones, but don't give up! Your options include switching to a medical provider who *is* knowledgeable about hormone balancing, contacting a compounding pharmacy for advice or referral, or consulting my Web site and educating yourself further. The Web site is set up for lab-result consultations and to order labs that are necessary after evaluating symptoms. (Please keep in mind that there is a fee for this service.)

Begin the treatment plan   Once you've established a treatment plan, continue it for 90 days.

Retest your levels   Retesting should be done at that same time in the cycle; if you're not cycling, order the tests after 90 days.

Adjust dosages   Make the necessary dosing adjustments to reach optimal ranges, then retest in four to six months.

The 12-Week Diet Overhaul

Weeks 1–2   Begin cleansing your body. Eliminate all sugar, flour, and dairy products for two weeks. Every day, drink eight to ten glasses of water and consume at least four to six servings of fruits and vegetables. Include ample amounts of protein and good, omega-rich fat, including almonds, olives or olive oil, fish oil, or flaxseed oil. Slow-cooked oatmeal is the only starch permitted during this initial phase of the diet.

Weeks 3–6   Reintroduce one to two starches per day and two dairy options. Do not include any white-flour products, but the following healthy options are permitted: sweet potatoes, brown rice (½-cup serving), sprouted-wheat bread (one slice), low-sugar yogurt, low-fat cheese or cream cheese, and 1 cup of low-fat or nonfat milk.

Weeks 6–12   You may continue to add back other dairy options and may take one full free day per week to eat anything you want. You can also reintroduce one free starch per day. I suggest that the starch be taken early in the day rather than in the evening.

Your ongoing diet will be modified between weeks 6 and 12, but should not vary dramatically. You are basically trying to eat more whole grains, proteins, beans and legumes, nuts, and whole, bright-colored fruits and vegetables. (But not sprinkle donuts!) When you eat this way, you will be amazed at how good you feel. You will drop fat from your midsection and experience renewed energy, better moods, and fewer cravings. Your hormonal balance will straighten out, and you will be back on track. If you go on vacation, eat all the wrong things, and feel horrible when you return, try revisiting the plan's first two weeks for at least 72 hours, and you will be back on track.

Remember that addictions to sugar, flour, and "zero" foods can be intense. You may need to detox from them more often than you think. Women's tolerance levels to empty calories vary. If you don't feel well while following the diet strictly and need to include a starch, use only sprouted-wheat bread and no other. If you crave chocolate every day after you have a free day, lighten up on the sugar on your free day. Know that when you eat sugar, you will crave it for the next three days. Is it worth it?

De-Stressing

All I need to say here is that you *must* do this. You will never lose weight and feel good without taking time for *you*. Reduce or eliminate caffeine and sugar and concentrate on conscious breathing all day long—deep, cleansing breaths. Take seriously the need to go for a walk, take a nap, soak in the tub after dinner, or walk around the block with your kids. You need to clear your head, work your body, and not take yourself so seriously. It will all be there when you return.

The Six-Step Plan for Jumpstarting Energy

Step 1   Exercise your body every day for at least 20 minutes.

Step 2   Add strength-training exercise three times per week for at least 30 minutes. This will build muscle, which is the best way I know to increase metabolism and energy.

Step 3   Add B-complex vitamins to your diet for necessary fuel, concentration, and memory.

Step 4   Eliminate excessive "bad fat" in your diet, which wears you down, makes you feel depressed, and zaps your energy. Kick the fast-food habit and appreciate a good piece of fresh fruit.

Step 5   Eat every three to four hours. Include protein and long-lasting carbohydrates, such as fruits and vegetables, and omega-rich fats like nuts and seeds.

Step 6   Stop worrying! Worry, anger, emotional distress, and irritability deplete you more than just about anything. In addition, stress takes years off your life and will most likely make everyone around you miserable, too.

You Can Do It

I think that this is enough to tackle in twelve weeks. I know that you are ready to take this on; otherwise, you would not have reached this point in the book! I challenge you to take this new course for your life. Making the commitment to improve your health is the first step toward a happier, healthier, longer life. I can honestly say that honoring these principles is the only way that I can accomplish my goals. And for so many of my patients, following a 12-week plan has been a complete life overhaul and nothing that they ever expected to happen.

Good luck on your journey! Please e-mail me (nj@nishajackson.com) about your progress. I would love to keep up on the positive changes that are taking place!

Appendix A

Compounding Pharmacies and Hormone-Testing Laboratories

Compounding Pharmacies

To find a compounding pharmacy near you, contact one of these professional associations:

International Academy of Compounding
Pharmacists (IACP)
P.O. Box 1365
Sugar Land, TX 77487
(800) 927-4227
www.iacprx.org

Professional Compounding Centers
of America, Inc. (PCCA)
9901 South Wilcrest
Houston, TX 77099
(800) 331-2498
www.pccarx.com

You can also contact any of these compounding pharmacies for help and referrals:

Marquis Compounding Pharmacy
4560 SE International Way, Suite 101
Milwaukie, OR 97222
(877) 542-4023
www.marquisrx.com

MedQuest Pharmacy
111 East 12300 South
Draper, UT 84020
(888) 222-2956
www.medquestpharmacy.com

Women's International Pharmacy
Arizona:
12012 North 111th Avenue
Youngtown, AZ 85363
(623) 214-7700

Wisconsin:
2 Marsh Court
Madison, WI 53718
(608) 221-7800
(800) 279-5708
www.womensinternational.com

Hormone-Testing Laboratories

AAL Reference Laboratories
1715 E. Wilshire Boulevard, Suite 715
Santa Ana, CA 92705
(800) 522-2611
www.antibodyassay.com

*This laboratory provides hormone testing
and a variety of other types of tests for
general well-being.*

Aeron Life Cycles
1933 Davis Street, Suite 310
San Leandro, CA 94577
(800) 631-7900
www.aeron.com

*This company tests for a panel of
hormones; available to consumers
and to medical providers.*

Doctors Data Inc. & Reference Laboratory
P.O. Box 111
West Chicago, IL 60185
(800) 323-2787
www.doctorsdata.com

This laboratory offers many tests, including blood, urine, and hair analysis.

Great Smokies Diagnostic Laboratory
63 Zillicoa Street
Asheville, NC 28801
(888) 891-3061
www.gsdl.com

This lab offers a variety of saliva testing for hormone analysis, as well as other tests, including for bowel health, allergies, and cardiovascular health.

Meridian Valley Clinical Laboratory
515 West Harrison Street, Suite 9
Kent, WA 98042
(800) 234-6285
www.meridianvalleylab.com

Full-range hormone analysis testing is available to both the consumer and the medical provider.

> *For testing laboratories in Canada, contact George Gillson, M.D., Ph.D., at Rocky Mountain Analytic Lab, (403) 241-4514.*

Rhein Consulting Laboratories
1175 SW Scholls Ferry Road, Suite 101
Portland, OR 97225
(503) 292-1988
www.rheinlabs.com

This laboratory offers hormone testing using the 24-hour urine method for measuring estrogens, progesterone, testosterone, DHEA, corticosteroids, and adrenal stress levels. It requires a prescription from your practitioner to whom the results will also be sent.

Southern Oregon Health and Wellness
3180 State Street, Suite 101
Medford, OR 97504
(541) 773-9772
www.southernoregonhealth.com

Consultation, testing, and recommendations for hormone treatment are available through the Web site and/or live phone calls.

ZRT Laboratory
12505 NW Cornell Road
Portland, OR 97213
(503) 469-0741
www.salivatest.com

Dr. David Zava is a biochemist who has done years of research on the effects of hormones on breast cells. His laboratory offers full-service saliva hormone analysis and blood spot testing.

Other Resources

American College for Advancement in Medicine (ACAM)
23121 Verdug Drive, Suite 204
Laguna Hills, CA 92653
(800) 532-3688
www.acam.org

For a referral to a practitioner who is knowledgeable about alternative medicine and the use of natural hormone replacement, you can contact the ACAM.

American Menopause Foundation
350 Fifth Avenue, Suite 2922
New York, NY 10118
(212) 714-2398
www.americanmenopause.org

This organization is dedicated to providing support and assistance on issues that surround menopause. The foundation has a newsletter available upon request.

Appendix B

Vitamin and Herbal Supplement Resources

Vitamin Deficiency Testing

This testing will determine if you are low in specific macronutrients or vitamins.

SpectraCell Laboratories, Inc.
7051 Port West, Suite 100
Houston, TX 77024
(800) 227-5227
www.spectracell.com

Vitamin and Herbal Supplements

Amazon Herb Company
1002 Jupiter Park Lane
Jupiter, FL 33458
(800) 835-0850
www.rainforestbio.com

This company specializes in products that enhance the effects of natural hormones or are used in place of hormones.

Beyond a Century
HC 76 Box 200
Greenville, ME 04441
(800) 777-1324
www.beyond-a-century.com

This company carries nutritional products, amino acids, antioxidants formulas, weight-loss formulas, and meal replacements.

Hahnemann's Laboratories
1940 4th Street
San Rafael, CA 94901
(888) 427-6422
www.hahnemannlabs.com

This laboratory has combination homeopathic remedies for specific hormonal symptoms.

Prevail
2204 NW Birdsdale
Gresham, OR 97030
(800) 248-0885
www.prevail.com

Natural plant enzyme products.

Rx Vitamins
200 Myrtle Boulevard
Larchmont, NY 10538
(800) 792-2222
www.rxvitamins.com

Distributed through medical providers.

Southern Oregon Health and Wellness, PC
3180 State Street, Suite 101
Medford, OR 97504
(541) 773-9772
www.southernoregonhealth.com

I created this Web site to help women identify supplements that are needed for different life stages and for specific hormonal problems. Free consultations on supplements are available. Testing for nutritional deficiencies or food allergies is also available with consultations.

Transitions for Health, Inc.
621 SW Alder Street, Suite 900
Portland, OR 97205
(800) 648-8211
www.transitionsforhealth.com

This company offers premium products, services, and informative materials on hormonal balancing for women. It is continuously developing products specifically for women in the area of wellness and vitality.

Vitamin Express
1428 Irving Street
San Francisco, CA 94122-2016
(415) 564-8160
www.vitaminexpress.com

This vitamin resource in the Bay Area is dedicated to offering a full spectrum of health foods and vitamins that they can mail to you.

Western Research Laboratories
21602 North 21st Avenue
Phoenix, AZ 85027
(877) 797-7997
www.westernrearchlaboratories.com

This is a resource for natural thyroid.

Appendix C

Products

Information on all of the products listed here can be obtained through www.southernoregonhealth.com or by calling (541) 773-9772.

Weight-Loss Supplements

- Weekly weight-loss packets
- Chromium picolinate
- L-carnitine
- Fat burners
- Essential fatty acids/flaxseed oil
- Thyroid-stimulating supplements
- Fat-burning protein shakes
- Fat-burning protein bars

Products for Sexual Dysfunction

- Eros Stimulator for improved sensation and blood flow
- Kegel Master for improved tone and improved incontinence
- Viagra cream for enhanced sensation
- Alvimil for sex drive
- Myself system for muscle strengthening
- L-argenine

Products for Treatment of PMS

- Full-spectrum light
- Weekly female balancing packets
- Evening primrose oil
- Progesterone cream
- 5-HTP supplement

Products for Treatment of Insomnia

- Melatonin drops (sublingual)
- 5-HTP supplement
- Valerian root

Products for Incontinence

- Kegel Master
- Myself system

Appendix D

Recommended Reading for Specific Perimenopausal Problems

Natural Hormones

Brown, Ellen, and Lynn Walker. *Menopause and Estrogen: Natural Alternatives to Hormone Replacement Therapy.* Berkeley, Calif.: Frog Ltd., 1996.

Laux, Marcus, and Christine Conrad. *Natural Woman, Natural Menopause.* New York: HarperCollins, 1997.

Lee, John R., and Virginia Hopkins. *What Your Doctor May Not Tell You About Menopause.* New York: Warner Books, 1996.

Northrup, Christiane. *The Wisdom of Menopause: Creating Physical and Emotional Health and Healing During the Change.* New York: Bantam Books, 2001.

Reiss, Uzzi, and Martin Zucker. *Natural Hormone Balance for Women.* New York: Pocket Books, 2001.

Schwartz, Erika. *The Hormone Solution: Naturally Alleviate Symptoms of Hormone Imbalance from Adolescence Through Menopause.* New York: Warner Books, 2002.

Vliet, Elizabeth Lee. *Screaming to Be Heard: Hormone Connections Women Suspect and Doctors Still Ignore.* New York: M. Evans and Company, 1995.

PMS and Depression

Cousens, Gabriel, and Mark Mayell. *Depression-Free for Life.* New York: HarperCollins, 2000.

Dalton, Katharina. *The Premenstrual Syndrome and Progesterone Therapy.* London: William Heinemann, 1984.

Lee, John R., David Zava, and Virginia Hopkins. *What Your Doctors May Not Tell You About Breast Cancer: How Hormone Balance Can Help Save Your Life.* New York: Warner Books, 2002

Schwartz, Erika. *The Hormone Solution: Naturally Alleviate Symptoms of Hormone Imbalance from Adolescence Through Menopause.* New York: Warner Books, 2002.

Vliet, Elizabeth Lee. "New Insights on Hormones and Mood." *Menopause Management* (June/July 1993): 14–16.

Ross, Julia. *The Diet Cure: The 8-Step Program to Rebalance Your Body Chemistry and End Food Cravings, Weight Problems, and Mood Swings—Now.* New York: Penguin Books, 2000.

Thyroid

The American Medical Women's Association. *The Women's Complete Guide to Wellness,* rev. ed. New York: Golden Books, 1998.

Brody, Jane E., et al. *The New York Times Guide to Alternative Health.* New York: Times Books, 2001.

Mayo, Mary Ann, and Joseph L. Mayo. *The Menopause Manager: A Safe Path for a Natural Change.* Grand Rapids: Fleming H. Revell, 1998.

Shames, Richard L., and Karilee Halo Shames. *Thyroid Power: Ten Steps to Total Health.* New York: HarperCollins, 2001.

Vliet, Elizabeth Lee. *Screaming to Be Heard: Hormone Connections Women Suspect and Doctors Still Ignore.* New York: M. Evans and Company, 1995.

Weight Loss and Nutrition and Exercise

Challem, Jack, Burton Berkson, and Melissa Diane Smith. *Syndrome X: The Complete Nutritional Program to Prevent and Reverse Insulin Resistance.* New York: John Wiley & Sons, 2000.

Colbert, Don, M.D. *What Would Jesus Eat? The Ultimate Program for Eating Well, Feeling Great, and Living Longer.* Nashville: Thomas Nelson, 2002.

Gillespie, Larrian. *The Menopause Diet.* Beverly Hills: Healthy Life Publications, 1999.

Mayo, Mary Ann, and Joseph L. Mayo. *The Menopause Manager: A Safe Path for a Natural Change.* Grand Rapids: Fleming H. Revell, 1998.

Neil, Kate, and Patrick Holford. *Balance Hormones Naturally.* Freedom, Calif.: The Crossing Press, 1999.

Perricone, Nicholas. *The Wrinkle Cure: Unlock the Power of Cosmeceuticals for Supple, Youthful Skin.* New York: Warner Books, 2000.

Peskin, Brian Scott. *Radiant Health: Moving Beyond the Zone.* Houston: Noble, 2001.

Phillips, Bill. *Body for Life: 12 Weeks to Mental and Physical Strength.* New York: HarperCollins, 1999.

Sears, Barry. *Enter The Zone.* New York: HarperCollins, 1995.

Smith, Pamela M. *Smart Weigh.* Washington, D.C.: LifeLine Press, 2002.

Eades, Michael, and Mary Dan Eades, *Protein Power: The High-Protein/Low-Carbohydrate Way to Lose Weight, Feel Fit, and Boost Your Health—In Just Weeks!* New York: Bantam, 1996.

Heller, Rachel, and Richard Heller. *The Carbohydrates Addict's Diet.* New York: Penguin Group, 1993.

Shealy, C. Norman. *DHEA: The Youth and Health Hormone.* New Canaan: Keats, 1996.

Stress Management

The Bible

Bost, Brent W. *The Hurried Woman.* New York: Vantage Press, 2001.

Foley, Denise, et al. *Women's Encyclopedia of Health and Emotional Healing.* Emmaus, Pa.: Rodale Press, 1993.

Komoroff, Anthony L. (ed.). *Harvard Medical School Family Health Guide.* New York: Simon & Schuster, 1999.

Lush, Jean, and Pam Vredevelt. *Women and Stress: A Practical Approach to Managing Tension.* Grand Rapids: Fleming H. Revell, 1992.

Northrup, Christiane. *Women's Bodies, Women's Wisdom.* New York: Bantam Books, 1994.

Spera, Stefanie, and Sandra Lanto. *Beat Stress with Strength: Achieving Wellness at Work and in Life.* New York: DBM Publishing, 1995.

Vliet, Elizabeth Lee. *Screaming to Be Heard: Hormone Connections Women Suspect and Doctors Still Ignore.* New York: M. Evans and Company, 1995.

Waterhouse, Debra. *Outsmarting Female Fatigue: Eight Energizing Strategies for Lifelong Vitality.* New York: Hyperion, 2001.

Menopause

Northrup, Christiane. *The Wisdom of Menopause: Creating Physical and Emotional Health and Healing During the Change.* New York: Bantam Books, 2001.

Reiss, Uzzi, and Martin Zucker. *Natural Hormone Balance for Women.* New York: Pocket Books, 2001.

Sex Drive

Berman, Jennifer, et al. *For Women Only: A Revolutionary Guide to Overcoming Sexual Dysfunction and Reclaiming Your Sex Life.* New York: Henry Holt, 2001.

Ferrare, Cristina. *Okay, So I Don't Have a Headache.* New York: St. Martin's/Griffin, 1999.

Maleskey, Gale, et al. *The Hormone Connection: Revolutionary Discoveries Linking Hormones and Women's Health Problems.* Emmaus, Pa.: Rodale Press, 2001.

Shealy, C. Norman. *DHEA: The Youth and Health Hormone.* New Canaan: Keats, 1996.

Sherwin, B. B., et al. "Androgen Enhances Sexual Motivation in Females: A Prospective, Crossover Study of Sex Steroid Administration in the Surgical Menopause. *Psychosomatic Medicine* 47 (1985): 339.

Young, Ronald L. "Androgens in Postmenopausal Therapy?" *Menopause Management* (May 1993): 21–24.

Vliet, Elizabeth Lee. *Screaming to Be Heard: Hormone Connections Women Suspect and Doctors Still Ignore.* New York: M. Evans and Company, 1995.

Appendix E

Bibliography

Chapter 1 – Why Hormonal Chaos?

Cone, Faye Kitchener. *Making Sense of Menopause.* New York: Simon & Schuster, 1993.

Laux, Marcus, and Christine Conrad. *Natural Woman, Natural Menopause.* New York: HarperCollins, 1997.

Lemon, Henry M., et al. "Reduced Estriol Excretion in Patients with Breast Cancer Prior to Endocrine Therapy." *Journal of the American Medical Association* (27 June 1966): 112–20.

Northrup, Christiane. *The Wisdom of Menopause: Creating Physical and Emotional Health and Healing During the Change.* New York: Bantam Books, 2001.

———. *Women's Bodies, Women's Wisdom.* New York: Bantam Books, 1994.

"Report of Cancer Incidence and Prevalence Projections," East Anglican Cancer Intelligence Unit, Department of Community Medicine, University of Cambridge, Macmillan Cancer Relief (June 1997).

Chapter 2 – Know Your Hormones in and out of Balance

Berne, Robert M., and Mathew N. Levy. "The Endocrine System: Mechanism of Action on Gonadal Steroid." *Physiology.* St. Louis: Mosby Co., 1983.

Brown, Ellen, and Lynn Walker. *Menopause and Estrogen: Natural Alternatives to Hormone Replacement Therapy.* Berkeley, Calif.: Frog Ltd., 1996.

Cowan, Linda D., et al. "Breast Cancer Incidence in Women with a History of Progesterone Deficiency." *American Journal of Epidemiology* 114.2 (1981): 209–17.

Glass, Robert H., Nathan G. Kase, and Leon Speroff. *Clinical Gynecological Endocrinology and Infertility,* 4th ed. Philadelphia: Williams & Wilkins, Inc., 1989.

Herman-Glidens, M. E., et al. "Secondary Sexual Characteristics and Menses in Young Girls Seen in Office Practice: A Study from the Pediatric Research in Office Settings Network." *Archives of Pediatric and Adolescent Medicine* 106 (3) (September 2000): 622–23.

Hertoghe, Thierry, and Jules-Jacques Nabet. *The Hormone Solution: Stay Younger Longer with Natural Hormone and Nutrition Therapies.* New York: Harmony Books, 2002.

Lee, John R., Jesse Hanley, and Virginia Hopkins. *What Your Doctor May Not Tell You About Premenopause: Balance Your Hormones and Your Life from Thirty to Fifty.* New York: Warner Books, 1999.

Maddox, Ronald W. "The New Science of Estrogen Receptors." *U.S. Pharmacist* (April 1999): 87–95.

Mashchak, Ann C., et al. "Comparison of Pharmacodynamic Properties of Various Estrogen Formulations." *American Journal of Obstetrics and Gynecology* (1 Nov. 1982): 511–18.

Mayo, Mary Ann, and Joseph L. Mayo. *The Menopause Manager: A Safe Path for a Natural Change.* Grand Rapids: Fleming H. Revell, 1998.

Chapter 3 – Have Your Hormones Tested

Berthonneau, J., et al. "Evolution of Salivary Estradiol Levels During the Spontaneous Menstrual Cycle: Correlation Between Saliva and Plasma." *Journal of Gynecologie, Obstetrique Et Biologie de la Reproduction* 18 (1989): 47–52.

Bralley, J. A., and R. S. Lord. *Laboratory Evaluations in Molecular Medicine: Nutrients Toxicants, and Cell Regulators.* Norcross, Ga.: Institute for Advances in Molecular Medicine, 2001.

Burrin, J. M., S. G. Johnson, and G. F. Joplin. "Direct Assay for Testosterone in Saliva: Relationship with a Direct Serum Free Testosterone Assay." *Clinica Chimica Acta* 163 (1987): 309–18.

Campbell, B. C., and P. T. Ellison. "Menstrual Variation in Salivary Testosterone Among Regularly Cycling Women." *Hormone Research* 37 (1992): 132–36.

Dabbs, James M. Jr. "Salivary Testosterone Measurements: Reliability Across Hours, Days, and Weeks." *Physiology and Behavior* 48 (1990): 83–86.

Finn, M. M., et al. "The Frequency of Salivary Progesterone Sampling and the Diagnosis of Luteal Phase Insufficiency." *Gynecological Endocrinology* 6 (1992): 127–34.

Finn, M. M., et al. "Follicular Growth and Corpus Luteum Function in Women with Unexplained Infertility, Monitored by Ultrasonography and Measurement of Daily Salivary Progesterone." *Gynecological Endocrinology* 3 (1989): 297–308.

Knyba, R. E., and D. Y. Wang. "Salivary Progesterone: Relation to Total and Non-Protein-Bound Blood Levels." *Journal of Steroid Biochemistry* 23 (1985): 975–79.

Kraemer, G., et.al., "Variability of Serum Estrogens Among Postmenopausal Women Treated with the Same Transdermal Estrogen Therapy and the Effect of Androgens and Sex Hormone Binding Globulin." *Fertility and Sterility* 79 (3) (March 2003).

Lee, John R., Jesse Hanley, and Virginia Hopkins. *What Your Doctor May Not Tell You About Premenopause: Balance Your Hormones and Your Life from Thirty to Fifty.* New York: Warner Books, 1999.

Maddox, Ronald W. "The New Science of Estrogen Receptors." *U.S. Pharmacist* (April 1999): 87–95.

McGinley, Robynne A., and Ross F. Vining. "The Measurement of Hormones in Saliva: Possibilities and Pitfalls." *Journal of Steroid Biochemistry* 27 (1987): 81–84.

Mounib, N., et al. "Correlations Between Free Plasma Estradiol and Estrogens Determined by Bioluminescence in Saliva, Plasma, and Urine During Spontaneous and FSH Stimulated Cycles in Women." *Journal of Steroid Biochemistry* 31 (1988): 861–65.

Nicolson, N., et al. "Salivary Cortisol Levels and Stress Reactivity in Human Aging." *Journal of Gerontology.* Series A, Biological Sciences and Medical Sciences 52 (1997): M68–75.

Northrup, Christiane. *The Wisdom of Menopause: Creating Physical and Emotional Health and Healing During the Change.* New York: Bantam Books, 2001.

———. *Women's Bodies, Women's Wisdom.* New York: Bantam Books, 1994.

Rouzier, Neal, and Cherie Constance. *Natural Hormone Replacement for Men and Women: How to Achieve Healthy Aging.* Salt Lake City: WorldLink Medical Publishing, 2001.

Sarrel, P., et al. "Estrogen and Estrogen-Androgen Replacement in Postmenopausal Women Dissatisfied with Estrogen and/or Androgen Administration in the Surgical Menopause." *American Journal of Obstetrics and Gynecology* 151 (1998): 153–60.

Swinkels, L. M., et al. "Concentrations of Total and Free Dehydroepiandrosterone in Plasma and Dehydroepiandrosterone in Saliva of Normal and Hirsute Women under Basal Conditions and During Administration of Dexamethasone/ Synthetic Corticotropin." *Clinical Chemistry* 36 (1990): 2042–46.

Vittek, Jozef, et al. "Direct Radioimmunoassay (RIA) of Salivary Testosterone: Correlation with Free and Total Serum Testosterone." *Life Sciences* 37 (1985): 711–16.

Vuorento, T., et al. "Daily Measurements of Salivary Progesterone Reveal a High Rate of Anovulation in Healthy Students." *Scandinavian Journal of Clinical and Laboratory Investigation* 49 (1989): 395–401.

Walker, R. F., et al. "Characterization of Profiles of Salivary Progesterone Concentrations During the Luteal Phase of Fertile and Subfertile Women." *Journal of Endocrinology* 104 (1985): 441–46.

Wang, D. Y., et al. "Salivary Oestradiol and Progesterone Levels in Premenopausal Women with Breast Cancer." *European Journal of Cancer and Clinical Oncology* 22 (1986): 427–33.

Wong, Y. F., et al. "Salivary Estradiol and Progesterone After In Vitro Fertilization and Embryo Transfer Using Different Luteal Support Regimens." *Reproduction, Fertility, and Development* 2 (1990): 351–58.

Wong, Y. F., et al. "Salivary Estradiol and Progesterone During the Normal Ovulatory Menstrual Cycle in Chinese Women." *European Journal of Gynecology and Reproductive Biology* 34 (1990): 129–35.

Chapter 4 – Use Hormones to Treat Hormone Problems

Anasti, J. N., H. B. Leonetti, and K. J. Wilson. "Topical Progesterone Cream Has Antiproliferative Effect on Estrogen-Stimulated Endometrium." *Obstetrics and Gynecology* 97 (April 2001): 4 supplement.

Burgess, A., J. Prior, M. Schechter, and Y. Vigna. "Spinal Bone Loss and Ovulatory Bone Disturbances." *New England Journal of Medicine*, vol. 323, no. 18, (1990): 122–7.

Cerhan, J. R., et al. "The Role of Hormone Replacement Therapy in the Risk for Breast Cancer and Total Mortality in Women with a Family History of Breast Cancer." *Annals of Internal Medicine* 127 (1997): 973–80.

Chang, King-Jen, Tigris T. Y. Lee, and Gustavo Lineres-Cruz. "Influences of Percutaneous Administration of Estradiol and Progesterone on Human Breast Epithelial Cell Cycle in Vivo." *Fertility and Sterility* 63.4 (1995): 785–91.

Dalton, Katharina. *The Premenstrual Syndrome and Progesterone Therapy*. London: William Heinemann, 1984.

Denesle, R., et al. "Sleep in Menopause: Differential Effects of Two Forms of Hormone Replacement Therapy." *Menopause: The Journal of The North American Menopause Society*, vol. 8, no. 1 (2001): 10–16.

Fraser, Ian S. *Estrogens and Progestogens in Clinical Practice*. London: Churchill Livingstone, 1998: 215–20.

Gambrell, R. D. Jr. "The True Impact of ERT in Menopause." *Hormone Therapy, The Complete Hormone Therapy Resource, American Health Consultants* (1999): 78–9.

Hargrove, Joel T., and Kevin G. Osteen. "An Alternative Method of Hormone Replacement Therapy Using the Natural Sex Steroids." *Infertility and Reproductive Medicine Clinics of North America* 6 (4) (1995): 653–74.

Hermsmeyer, K., et al. "Medroxyprogesterone Interferes with Ovarian Steroid Protection Against Coronary Vasospasm." *Natural Medicine*, vol. 3, no. 3 (March 1997): 324–27.

Hudson, Tori. *Women's Encyclopedia of Natural Medicine*. Lincolnwood, Ill.: Keats, 1999.

Mashchak, Ann C., et al. "Comparison on Pharmacodynamic Properties of Various Estrogen Formulations." *American Journal of Obstetrics and Gynecology* (1 Nov. 1982): 511–18.

Maxson, W. S. "The Use of Progesterone in the Treatment of PMS." *Clinical Obstetrics and Gynecology* 30 (1987): 465–77.

Reiss, Uzzi, and Martin Zucker. *Natural Hormone Balance for Women.* New York: Pocket Books, 2001.

Rouzier, Neal, and Cherie Constance. *Natural Hormone Replacement for Men and Women: How to Achieve Healthy Aging.* Salt Lake City: WorldLink Medical Publishing, 2001.

Rudel, H. W., and F. A. Sind. "Toxicity of Progesterone." *International Encyclopedia of Pharmacology and Therapeutics.* New York: Pergamon Press, 1991.

Vliet, Elizabeth Lee. *Screaming to Be Heard: Hormone Connections Women Suspect and Doctors Still Ignore.* New York: M. Evans and Company, 1995.

Wright, Jonathan V., and John Morgenthaler. *Natural Hormone Replacement.* Petaluma, Calif.: Smart, 1997.

Writers' Group for the Women's Health Initiative Investigators. "Risks and Benefits of Estrogen plus Progestin in Healthy Postmenopausal Women: Principal Results from the Women's Health Initiative Randomized Controlled Trial." *Journal of the American Medical Association* 288 (2002): 321–333.

Young, Ronald L. "Androgens in Postmenopausal Therapy?" *Menopause Management* (May 1993): 21–24.

Chapter 5 – Fix Your Diet: The Most Powerful Way to Create Hormonal Balance

Challem, Jack, Burton Berkson, and Melissa Diane Smith. *Syndrome X: The Complete Nutritional Program to Prevent and Reverse Insulin Resistance.* New York: John Wiley & Sons, 2000.

Chmouliovsky, L., et al. "Beneficial Effect of Hormone Replacement Therapy on Weight Loss in Obese Menopausal Women." *Maturitas* 32 (3) (1999): 148–52.

De Pergola, G., et al. "Body Fat Accumulation Is Possibly Responsible for Lower Dehydroepiandrosterone Circulating Levels in Premenopausal Obese Women." *International Journal of Obesity Related Metabolic Disorders* 20 (12) (1996): 1105–10.

Duncan, K. H., et al. "Effect of Low-Calorically Dense (LCD) vs. High-Calorically Dense (HCD) Diets in Non-Obese and Obese People." *American Journal of Nutrition* 37 (1999): 763–767.

Gillespie, Larrian. *The Menopause Diet.* Beverly Hills: Healthy Life Publications, 1999.

Heller, Rachel, and Richard Heller. *The Carbohydrates Addict's Diet.* New York: Penguin Group, 1993.

Mayo, Mary Ann, and Joseph L. Mayo. *The Menopause Manager: A Safe Path for a Natural Change.* Grand Rapids: Fleming H. Revell, 1998.

Neil, Kate, and Patrick Holford. *Balance Hormones Naturally.* Freedom, Calif.: The Crossing Press, 1999.

Perricone, Nicholas. *The Wrinkle Cure: Unlock the Power of Cosmeceuticals for Supple, Youthful Skin.* New York: Warner Books, 2000.

Peskin, Brian Scott. *Radiant Health: Moving Beyond the Zone.* Houston: Noble, 2001.

Sears, Barry. *Enter The Zone.* New York: HarperCollins, 1995.

Shealy, C. Norman. *DHEA: The Youth and Health Hormone.* New Canaan: Keats, 1996.

Smith, Pamela M. *Take Charge of the Change.* Grand Rapids: Zondervan, 2003.

Waterhouse, Debra. *Outsmarting the Midlife Fat Cell: Winning Weight Control Strategies for Women over 35 to Stay Fit Through Menopause.* New York: Hyperion, 1999.

Chapter 6 – Eliminate the Stress Hormone

Bost, Brent W. *The Hurried Woman.* New York: Vantage Press, 2001.

Foley, Denise, et al. *Women's Encyclopedia of Health and Emotional Healing.* Emmaus, Pa.: Rodale Press, 1993.

Friedenreich, C. M. "Physical Activity and Cancer Prevention: From Observational to Intervention Research." *Cancer Epidemiology Biomarkers Prevention* 10 (2001): 287–301.

Komoroff, Anthony L. (ed.). *Harvard Medical School Family Health Guide.* New York: Simon & Schuster, 1999.

Lush, Jean, and Pam Vredevelt. *Women and Stress: A Practical Approach to Managing Tension.* Grand Rapids: Fleming H. Revell, 1992.

Northrup, Christiane. *Women's Bodies, Women's Wisdom.* New York: Bantam Books, 1994.

Pert, Candace B. *Molecules of Emotion: The Science Behind Mind-Body Medicine.* New York: Touchstone Books, 1997: 191–193.

Spera, Stefanie, and Sandra Lanto. *Beat Stress with Strength: Achieving Wellness at Work and in Life.* New York: DBM Publishing, 1995.

Vliet, Elizabeth Lee. *Screaming to Be Heard: Hormone Connections Women Suspect and Doctors Still Ignore.* New York: M. Evans and Company, 1995.

Waterhouse, Debra. *Outsmarting Female Fatigue: Eight Energizing Strategies for Lifelong Vitality.* New York: Hyperion, 2001.

Chapter 7 – Get a Grip on PMS

Cousens, Gabriel, and Mark Mayell. *Depression-Free for Life.* New York: HarperCollins, 2000.

Dalton, Katharina. *The Premenstrual Syndrome and Progesterone Therapy.* London: William Heinemann, 1984.

Ford, Gillian. *Listening to Your Hormones.* Rockville, Calif.: Prima Publishing, 1997.

Holick, M. F. McCollum Award Lecture: "Vitamin D: New Horizons for the Twenty-first Century. *American Journal of Clinical Nutrition* 60 (1994): 619–30.

Maleskey, Gale, et al. *The Hormone Connection: Revolutionary Discoveries Linking Hormones and Women's Health Problems.* Emmaus, Pa.: Rodale Press, 2001.

Maxson, W. S. "The Use of Progesterone in the Treatment of PMS." *Clinical Obstetrics and Gynecology* 30 (1987): 465–77.

Norris, R.V. "Progesterone for Premenstrual Tension." *Journal of Reproductive Medicine* 8 (1983): 509–16.

Rosenthal, Norman E. *Winter Blues: Seasonal Affective Disorder: What It Is and How to Overcome It.* New York: Guilford Press, 1998.

Schechter, Dianne. "Estrogen, Progesterone, and Mood." *Journal of Gender-Specific Medicine* 2 (1999): 29–36.

Smith, Pamela M. *Take Charge of the Change.* Grand Rapids: Zondervan, 2003.

Vliet, Elizabeth Lee. "New Insights on Hormones and Mood." *Menopause Management* (June/July 1993): 14–16.

———. *Screaming to Be Heard: Hormone Connections Women Suspect and Doctors Still Ignore.* New York: M. Evans and Company, 1995.

Women's Nutritional Advisory Service. "Social Implications of Premenstrual Syndrome: 11 Years On" (1996).

Chapter 8 – Turn On Your Sex Drive

Berman, Jennifer, et al. *For Women Only: A Revolutionary Guide to Overcoming Sexual Dysfunction and Reclaiming Your Sex Life.* New York: Henry Holt, 2001.

Ferrare, Cristina. *Okay, So I Don't Have a Headache.* New York: St. Martin's/Griffin, 1999.

Guay, A. T. "Decreased Testosterone in Regularly Menstruating Women with Decreased Libido: A Clinical Observation." *Journal of Sex Marital Therapy* 27 (5) (2001): 513–18.

Maleskey, Gale, et al. *The Hormone Connection: Revolutionary Discoveries Linking Hormones and Women's Health Problems.* Emmaus, Pa.: Rodale Press, 2001.

Rako, Susan. *The Hormone Desire: The Truth About Sexuality, Menopause, and Testosterone.* New York: Three Rivers Press, 1999.

Shealy, C. Norman. *DHEA: The Youth and Health Hormone.* New Canaan: Keats, 1996.

Shifren, J. L., et al. "Transdermal Testosterone Treatment in Women with Impaired Sexual Function after Oophorectomy." *New England Journal of Medicine* 343 (2000): 682–88.

Young, Ronald L. "Androgens in Postmenopausal Therapy?" *Menopause Management* (May 1993): 21–24.

Vliet, Elizabeth Lee. *Screaming to Be Heard: Hormone Connections Women Suspect and Doctors Still Ignore.* New York: M. Evans and Company, 1995.

Chapter 9 – The Fatigue Factor: Rejuvenate Your Thyroid

Adlin, Victor. "Subclinical Hypothyroidism: Deciding When to Treat." *American Family Physician Magazine* (15 February 1998).

Arem, R. *The Thyroid Solution: A Mind-Body Program for Beating Depression and Regaining Your Emotional and Physical Health.* New York: Ballantine Books, 1999.

Barnes, Broda O., and Lawrence Galton. *Hypothyroidism: The Unsuspected Illness.* New York: Harper and Row, 1976.

Barnes, B. "Basal Temperature Versus Basal Metabolism." *Journal of American Medical Association* 119 (1942): 1073–74.

Brody, Jane E., et al. *The New York Times Guide to Alternative Health.* New York: Times Books, 2001.

Canaris, G. J., et al. "The Colorado Thyroid Disease Prevalence Study." *Archives of Internal Medicine* 160 (2000): 526–34.

Danese, M. D., et al. "Screening for Mild Thyroid Failure in the Periodic Health Examination: A Decision and Cost-Effective Analysis." *Journal of American Medical Association* 276 (1996): 285–92.

Hak, E., et al. "Subclinical Hypothyroidism Is an Independent Risk Factor for Atherosclerosis and Myocardial Infarction in Elderly Women: The Rotterdam Study." *Annuals of Internal Medicine* 132 (4) (2000): 691–97.

Larsen, P. R., and S. H. Ingbar. "The Thyroid Gland," in *Textbook of Endocrinology*, 8th ed., J. F. Wilson, and D. W. Foster (eds.) Philadelphia: W. B. Saunders, 1992: 357–487.

Lopez, A., et al. "The Risk Factors and Bone Mineral Density in Women in Long-Term Levothyroxine Treatment." *Medical Clinics* (Barcelona) 112, no. 3 (1999): 85–89.

Mayo, Mary Ann, and Joseph L. Mayo. *The Menopause Manager: A Safe Path for a Natural Change.* Grand Rapids: Fleming H. Revell, 1998.

Nuzzo, V., et al. "Bone Mineral Density in Premenopausal Women Receiving Levothyroxine Suppressive Therapy." *Gynecological Endocrinology* 12, no. 5 (1998): 333–37.

Ridgeway, E. C. *Hypothyroidism: The Hidden Challenge.* Monograph. University of Colorado School of Medicine, December 1996.

Shames, Richard L., and Karilee Halo Shames. *Thyroid Power: Ten Steps to Total Health.* New York: HarperCollins, 2001.

Skinner, G., et al. "Thyroxine Should Be Tried in Clinically Hypothyroid but Biochemically Euthyroid Patients." *British Medical Journal* 314 (1997): 1764–65.

Teitelbaum, Jacob. *From Fatigued to Fantastic!: A Proven Program to Regain Vibrant Health, Based on a New Scientific Study Showing Effective Treatment for Chronic Fatigue and Fibromyalgia.* New York: Avery, 2001.

The American Medical Women's Association. *The Women's Complete Guide to Wellness,* rev. ed. New York: Golden Books, 1998.

Vliet, Elizabeth Lee. *Screaming to Be Heard: Hormone Connections Women Suspect and Doctors Still Ignore.* New York: M. Evans and Company, 1995.

Chapter 10 – Other Hazards of Perimenopause

Aksa, M. F., R. B. Greenblatt, and V. A. Tzinquonis. "Estriol in the Management of Menopause." *Journal of the American Medical Association* 239 (1978).

Anasti, J. N., H. B. Leonetti, and K. J. Wilson. "Topical Progesterone Cream Has Antiproliferative Effect on Estrogen-Stimulated Endometrium." *Obstetrics and Gynecology* 97 (April 2001): 4 supplement.

Birge, S. J. "Hormones and the Aging Brain." *Geriatrics* 53 (suppl. I) (1998): S28–30.

Brown, J., and R. Tan. "Cognition and Estrogens in the Elderly Woman." *Clinical Geriatrics,* vol. 6, no. 5 (May 1998): 10–19.

Burgess, A., J. Prior, M. Schechter, and Y. Vigna. "Spinal Bone Loss and Ovulatory Bone Disturbances." *New England Journal of Medicine,* vol. 323, no. 18 (1990): 122–7.

Denesle, R., et al. "Sleep in Menopause: Differential Effects of Two Forms of Hormone Replacement Therapy." *Menopause: The Journal of The North American Menopause Society,* vol. 8, no. 1 (2001): 10–16.

Gambrell R. D. Jr. "The True Impact of ERT in Menopause." *Hormone Therapy, The Complete Hormone Therapy Resource, American Health Consultants* (1999): 78–9.

Goldstein, Steven R., and Laurie Ashner. *The Estrogen Alternative.* New York: G. P. Putnam's Sons, 1998.

Lemon, Henry M., et al. "Reduced Estriol Excretion in Patients with Breast Cancer Prior to Endocrine Therapy." *Journal of the American Medical Association* (27 June 1966): 112–20.

Rako, Susan. *The Hormone Desire: The Truth About Sexuality, Menopause, and Testosterone.* New York: Three Rivers Press, 1999.

Simpkins, J. W., et al. "Role of Estrogen Replacement Therapy in Memory Enhancement and the Prevention of Neuronal Loss Associated with Alzheimer's Disease." *American Journal of Medicine* 103 (3A) (1997): 19S-25S.

Glossary

5-HTP A supplement that acts as a precursor to the neurotransmitter serotonin; has been shown to be an effective supplement in the treatment of PMS, depression, insomnia, and weight control.

alopecia Early hair loss; an absence of hair from skin areas where it is normally present.

androgens A class of sex hormones associated with the development and maintenance of secondary sex characteristics and sexual differentiation. In addition to increasing sexual function and libido, they stimulate skeletal growth.

aphrodisiacs Foods that enhance sexual desire.

bi-estrogen Dual natural estrogen that incorporates two types of estrogen— estriol and estradiol; it matches the molecular structure of human estrogens.

bioidentical hormones Compounds that are formed to be molecularly identical to the hormones found in the patient's own body; they are quite different from many commercially marketed medications.

CBC Stands for *complete blood count.*

chronic fatigue syndrome An unusual illness of uncertain cause that typically presents as fatigue, weakness, muscle pain, lymph node swelling, and malaise.

circadian rhythm The "body clock" that regulates our sleep pattern; it tells us when to sleep, awaken, have a bowel movement, and be at our peak performance. Also regulates specific hormones in the body.

cortisol The stress hormone. Produced by the adrenal system in response to stress that can exert great influence on the nervous system, blood pressure, pulse rate, metabolism, and fat storage.

day 1 The first day of your period.

DHEA Stands for *dehydroepiandrosterone.* The most abundant of the sex steroids produced by the adrenal glands and to a lesser extent by the ovaries. A precursor to other sex hormones such as testosterone and estrogen. Helps the body's resistance to stress and disease. Appears to have a protective effect on the bones and the heart. A balancer to cortisol. Aides in brain function and energy.

DHEA-S Stands for *dehydroepiandrosterone-sulfate.* An androgen that is produced by the adrenal glands and the ovaries.

DIM Stands for *di-indolylmethane.*

endometriosis A condition in which tissue from the lining of the uterus, or similar tissue resembling the uterine mucous membrane (endometrium), occurs in various locations in the pelvic cavity, outside the uterine walls.

endorphins A morphinelike substance that kills pain and contributes to feelings of improved self-esteem, euphoria, and emotional well-being. The feel-good brain chemicals that are released during exercise; they counterbalance the ill effects of headaches.

EPO Stands for *evening primrose oil.*

estradiol The most potent of the estrogens and the one in greatest evidence in premenopausal women. Produced by fertile ovaries.

estriol The weakest form of the estrogens; it's at its highest levels during pregnancy. Produced from the conversion of estrone.

estrogen A key sex hormone primarily produced by the ovaries before menopause. It is the hormone that makes women feminine. Also maintains blood-sugar levels and protects against many diseases. Three types of estrogen are produced by the ovaries and, to a lesser extent, by the adrenal glands: *estradiol, estrone,* and *estriol.*

estrogen dominance The condition in which a woman's estrogen levels may be low, normal, or excessive, but she has little or no progesterone to balance the effects of estrogen on the body. Symptoms include weight gain, fibrocystic breasts, fibroid uterine tumors, unstable emotions, irritabil-ity, acne, and bloating. Menstrual irregularities such as heavy periods, cramping, or missed periods can also result.

estrone An estrogen produced from the conversion of estradiol in the fat cells. The dominant estrogen after menopause; associated with fat storage.

evening primrose oil (EPO) A supplement available in capsule form that can be effective for treating PMS.

fibrocystic breast disease Benign breast disease that presents as tiny, painful breast lumps that come and go with the cycle; closely related to estrogen and progesterone balance.

fibroids Benign smooth muscle tumors of the uterus that may cause vaginal bleeding and increased uterine cramping. The size of fibroids is driven largely by estrogen levels in the body.

follicular phase The preovulatory phase of the menstrual cycle, during which the follicle (egg) grows and high estrogen levels build up the uterine lining. Days 1 to 13 of the cycle. See also *proliferative phase.*

FSH Stands for *follicle-stimulating hormone.* Produced by the pituitary gland in the brain and stimulates the development of ovarian follicles (eggs) and the release of estrogen from the ovaries.

FSH test A blood test that can indicate the onset of menopause.

g Stands for *gram.*

globulin A category of blood proteins.

hormone panel Comprehensive test that that measures a woman's levels of estrogen, progesterone, testosterone, DHEA (dehydroepiandrosterone), and thyroid hormones.

hormone replacement therapy (HRT)
A prescribed hormone plan that may include estrogen, progesterone, and testosterone.

HRT See *hormone replacement therapy.*

hyperthyroidism Excessive functional activity of the thyroid gland, resulting in an overproduction of thyroid hormones.

hypothalamus A cherry-sized region of the brain that indirectly controls the release of numerous hormones, including sex hormones. It regulates body temperature, certain metabolic processes, and other autonomic activities.

hypothyroidism A condition resulting from underproduction of thyroid hormones from the thyroid glands, also known as *underactive thyroid.* Affects more women than men, and the risk increases with age for both. Symptoms include cold hands and feet, emotional disturbances, extreme fatigue, and constipation.

hysterectomy The surgical removal of part or all of the uterus.

I3C Stands for *indole-3-carbinol.*

insulin resistance Elevated insulin levels. A condition in which insulin, a fat-storage hormone, is constantly released in response to a high-sugar or high-processed-carbohydrate diet. Also a syndrome that is a precursor to diabetes.

isoflavones A type of phytoestrogen that has weak estrogenic activity. Isoflavones possess myriad biological properties that can affect many physiological processes and may help create a more balanced hormonal state. Isoflavones are found in chick-

peas and legumes and are most concentrated in soy.

IU Stands for *international units.*

Kegel exercises Pelvic muscle exercises—a simple tightening and releasing of the vaginal muscles (as if you were stopping urination). Also help strengthen the pelvic muscles to enhance orgasms, improve sexual sensation, and lubrication; can reduce incontinence-related problems.

levo-thyroxine See *T4.*

luteal phase The postovulatory phase of the menstrual cycle; the time in which progesterone is predominantly produced, causing the uterine lining to secrete substances that support the implantation of the embryo. Days 14 to 28 of the cycle. See also *secretory phase.*

mcg Stands for *microgram.*

melatonin The light-sensitive, sleep-regulating hormone produced by the pineal gland.

menopause The time when a woman's periods cease.

menstrual phase The phase of the menstrual cycle during which the lining of the uterus is shed (the first day of menstrual flow is considered day 1 of the menstrual cycle).

mg Stands for *milligram.*

MRI Stands for *magnetic resonance imaging* scan.

natural hormones Hormones in their purest form—bioidentical in molecular structure to those made by the human body. They have the same effect as the body's own hormones and do not interfere with the body's own hormone production.

ng/dl Stands for *nanograms per deciliter.*

oophorectomy The surgical removal of one or both ovaries.

ovulation The release, typically between days 12 and 14 of the menstrual cycle, of a single, mature egg that has developed in the ovary. Once it makes its way down the reproduction tract to the uterus, the egg can be fertilized for up to 48 hours before it begins to reabsorb.

osteoporosis A disease in which the bones become extremely porous, are subject to fracture, and heal slowly; occurs especially in women following menopause.

perimenopause The years leading up to menopause—usually between the ages of thirty-five and fifty—during which hormones fluctuate and birth control pills or hormone replacement therapy (HRT) may be prescribed. Symptoms include mood swings, depression, hot flashes, insomnia, weight gain, fatigue, and low sex drive.

pg/ml Stands for *picograms per milliliter.*

phytoestrogens Plant hormones.

PMS See *premenstrual syndrome.*

polycystic ovarian syndrome (PCOS) An endocrine disorder in any age group that disrupts the normal ovary cycles and often causes infertility. Many tiny cysts line the walls of the ovary that can interrupt normal hormonal processes, often resulting in high testosterone and insulin levels, with a disruption in the balance of estrogen and progesterone. Symptoms include facial hair, weight gain, acne, and depression.

PCOS See *polycystic ovarian syndrome.*

premenstrual syndrome Commonly known as *PMS.* Condition that includes physical and psychological/emotional symptoms associated with the later phase of the menstrual cycle. It is usually followed by a period of time that is symptom-free. Mood-related symptoms include irritability, depression, and fatigue. Physical symptoms include headaches, food cravings, water retention, breast tenderness, acne, hives, cold sores, herpes outbreaks, asthma, throat or gland swelling, seizures, recurrent yeast or bladder infections, and flu-like symptoms.

progesterone A hormone produced in the second half of the menstrual cycle after ovulation; works with estrogen to prepare the uterus for conception.

progestin A synthetic imitation of progesterone.

proliferative phase The phase of the menstrual cycle following menstruation, during which the pituitary gland, under the effect of FSH (follicle-stimulating hormone) from the ovary, makes estrogen, causing the lining of the uterus to thicken. The end of the proliferative phase is with the release of the egg (ovulation). See also *follicular phase.*

SAD Stands for *seasonal affective disorder.*

saliva test A salivary analysis of the hormone profile.

seasonal affective disorder (SAD) Psychological disorder caused by a lack of sunlight. Treated with full-spectrum light therapy.

secretory phase The second half of the menstrual cycle after ovulation; the corpus luteum secretes progesterone, which prepares the endometrium for the implantation of an embryo; if fertilization does not occur, menstrual flow will begin. See also *luteal phase.*

serotonin A chemical neurotransmitter that brings calm feelings of well-being. The brain chemical that may be associated with weight and depression control.

serum (blood) test Method of measuring the specified levels in the blood.

SHBG Stands for *sex hormone–binding globulin.* A protein that binds up testosterone.

sluggish liver A condition of the liver that may cause sluggishness in the detoxification process with hormonal balance. Aging, caffeine, sugar, alcohol, and medications that impair liver function can reduce the elimination of excessive estrogen.

Steroid hormones Cortisol, DHEA, estrogen, progesterone, and testosterone.

subclinical hypothyroidism An early state of an underactive thyroid condition.

sublingual Under the tongue.

T3 Stands for *triiodothyronine.* A short-acting thyroid hormone that controls energy in the body; more potent than T4.

T4 Stands for *levo-thyroxine.* A thyroid hormone that is carried in the circulation bound to protein. It is slow acting and referred to as the storage hormone.

testosterone Known as the forgotten hormone, especially in menopause. Present in both men and women, it is produced in small amounts by the ovaries and the adrenal glands. It is a vital hormone that women rely on for energy, vitality, sex drive, and endurance.

thyroid A butterfly-shaped gland at the front of the neck that extends to both sides of the Adam's apple. The thyroid gland controls every chemical reaction of nearly every organ in the body. Without it the body would cool off and slow down to the point of death.

topical On the skin.

toxic stress A condition in which a woman is under excessive and prolonged stress; the body churns out a poisonous level of stress hormones, which is too much to withstand on a day-to-day basis.

TRH Stands for *thyroid-releasing hormone.*

tri-estrogen Estrogen supplement that incorporates all three types of estrogen—estriol, estradiol, and estrone—but has the greatest amount of estriol.

triiodothyronine See *T3.*

TSH Stands for *thyroid-stimulating hormone.*

urine hormone test A type of testing that utilizes the urine to analyze hormone levels in the body.

vaginal/vulvar atrophy A thinning of the vaginal tissues; leads to problems with bladder control, lubrication, and vaginal infections such as yeast and bacteria overgrowth. Treatment improves tissue health and increases the area's elasticity, moistness, and padding.

xenohormones An element from outside the human body that performs a hormonelike communication inside the body. Xenohormones have been implicated in breast cancer development and many other illnesses.

Index

5-HTP, 95, 139

ACAM, 148
Adrenal glands, 77
Adrenal hormones, 77
Adrenal/liver support supplements, 106
Adrenal support supplements, 82
Aerobic activity, 69
Aging, 10–12, 62–64
Alcohol, 124, 139
Aldactone, 58, 130
Alopecia, 129
Alpha lipoic acid, 56, 128
American College for Advancement in
    Medicine (ACAM), 148
American Menopause Foundation, 148
Android, 102
Anti-androgen, 58
Antidepressants, 96
Aphrodisiacs, 100
Arem, Ridha, 110
Armour, 119
Astro-glide, 134
Atrophic changes, 133

B-complex, 82, 95, 120, 130
Baked potatoes, 65
Beals, Norman, Jr., 90
Beals, Norman, Sr., 90
Berman, Jennifer, 101
Bi-estrogen, 52–53, 126
Bibliography, 155–163
Bioidentical progesterone, 55

Biotin, 130
Birth control pills
    estrogen alternatives, as, 54
    estrogen dominance and, 22
    hair loss, 131
Black cohosh, 125
Bladder control, 137–138
    products, 151
Bloating, 93
Body image, 105, 107
Body weight. *See also* Diet
    aging, 62–64
    breast tenderness, 133
    estrogen imbalance, 55
    hair loss, 130
    products, 151
    supplements, 71
Body temperature, 117, 125, 139
Braunstein, Glenn D., 103
Breakfast, 70, 80, 81
Breast, anatomy, 132
Breast tenderness, 131–133
Breathing exercises, 83, 86
Busy women, 77–80. *See also* Working
    women

Caffeine, 137, 139
Calcium, 94
Calcium d-glucarate, 55
Calcium-magnesium, 82, 126, 139
Carbohydrates, 115
Cayenne peppers, 100
CBC, 113
Champagne, 100

Chilies, 100

Chocolate, 93, 100

Choline, 56

Chronic fatigue, 119

Chromium picolinate, 71, 120

Circadian rhythm, 138

Circulation enhancer, 104

Citrus vinaigrette, 67

Co-enzyme Q10, 71

Colorado Thyroid Disease Prevalence Study, 110

Complete blood count (CBC), 133

Complex carbohydrates, 115

Compounding pharmacies, 147

Copper, 120

Cranberry tablets, 93

Crunches, 105

Cysteine, 128

Cytomel, 119

D-alpha tocopherol, 120

Dairy products, 64

Dalton, Katharina, 89

De-stressing, 86, 144

Definitions (glossary), 164–168

Depression, 115, 119

DHEA, 103

DHEA-S, 129, 136, 139

Di-indolylmethane (DIM), 56, 128

Diet, 61–73

12-week diet overhaul, 143–144

aphrodisiacs, 100

breast tenderness, 132–133

estrogen dominance, 22

estrogen imbalance, 55

exercise, 69

fat, 68

fatigue, 115

fruits and vegetables, 66–67

hair loss, 129

hypoglycemia, 94

PMS, 91

protein, 64–65

six-step plan, 64–69

stress, 85

sugar, 65

supplements. *See* Supplements

tips for success, 69–70

water, 68

Dosage

estradiol, 37

estrogen, 53

progesterone, 37, 47–48

testosterone, 37, 59

Dream date at home, 108

Eat regularly, 70, 136

Endorphins, 136

Energy, 144

Enter the Zone (Sears), 62

EPO capsules, 94, 126

Epperson, Neill, 88

Eros Stimulator, 104, 151

Essential fatty acids, 133

Est-Pro, 96

Estradiol, 20, 36–38, 52, 103

Estratest, 102

Estriol, 20, 52, 103, 137

Estriol vaginal cream, 134

Estrogen, 19–22, 50–55

aging, 10

dosage, 53

hair loss, 131

hot flashes/night sweats, 126

imbalance, 54–55

natural choices, 52–53

periods, and, 54

sex drive, and, 100

synthetic alternatives, 53–54

too high/low, 21

vaginal dryness, 133–134

Estrogen deficiency, 133

Estrogen dominance, 18, 21–22

Estrogen patch, 53, 96, 126

Estrone, 20, 52

Evening primrose oil (EPO), 94, 126

Evening snacking, 70

Exercise

benefits, 72–73

bladder control, 137–138

breast tenderness, 130

fatigue, 115

headaches, 136

hot flashes/night sweats, 125

irregular bleeding, 128

sex drive, 104, 105
sleep, 139
stress, 80, 86
weight loss, 69
working women, 81

Fat, 68
Fatigue, 109–121
  causes, 113–115
  quick-fix plan for energy, 121
  supplements, 120
  testing, 116–117
  thyroid, 110–113
  treatment, 118–121
Fertility and Sterility, 30
Fiber, 128
Fibrocystic breast disease, 9
Fibroids, 9–10
Fibromyalgla, 119
5-HTP, 95, 139
Flaxseed, 120
Flaxseed oil, 126
Flaxseed oil capsules, 71
Flaxseed oil supplements, 128
Food. *See* Diet
Food diary, 69
Food supplements. *See* Supplements
Frequent meals, 70, 136
Friendship, 80, 83
Fruit, 66–67
Further reading, 152–154

GF Thyroid, 119
Gillson, George, 148
Ginger, 100
Ginseng, 71
Glossary, 164–168

Hair loss, 129–131
Headaches, 134–136
Healthcare provider, 38–39
Herbal supplements, 95, 149–150.
  See also Supplements
Herbed vinaigrette, 67
High-carbohydrate diet, 63
High-fiber diet, 55
High-protein, healthy snacks, 65

High-protein, low-fat snacks, 65
Hormonal blood test, 127–128
Hormonal domino effect, 18
Hormone Connection, The (Epperson), 88
Hormone cream, 137
Hormone Desire: The Truth About Sexuality, Menopause, and Testosterone, The (Rako), 102
Hormone-related headaches, 135–136
Hormone roller coaster, 8–10
Hormone testing, 2–3, 27–39
  interpreting lab results, 34–38
  saliva testing, 34, 35
  serum testing, 31–33
  timing, 31
  urine testing, 34
Hormone-testing laboratories, 147–148
Hormones, 41–59
  adrenal, 77
  estrogen. *See* Estrogen
  individualizing treatment, 44–45
  natural vs. synthetic, 42–44
  progesterone. *See* Progesterone
  sex drive, 101–103
  sleep-promoting, 139–140
  testosterone. *See* Testosterone
  thyroid, 116
  12-week hormonal overhaul, 142–143
Hot flashes, 124–127
Hyperthyroidism, 115
Hypoglycemia diet, 94
Hypothalamus, 99, 110
Hypothyroidism, 110–113. *See also* Fatigue
Hysterectomy, 22

Incontinence (bladder control), 137–138
Individualizing hormone treatment, 44–45
Indole-3-carbinol (I3C), 56, 128
Inositol, 56
Insomnia (sleep), 114–115, 138–140
Insulin resistance, 62, 63, 129
Iodine, 112
Iron-deficiency anemia, 113–114
Irregular bleeding, 127–128

K-Y Jelly, 134
Kegel exercises, 104, 137–138
Kegel Master, 104, 138, 151

Kelp, 120
Kenolog spray, 130

L-arginine, 105
L-carnitine, 71
L-glutamine, 71
L-tyrosine, 95
Label, 70
Lean proteins, 64
Lee, John, 21
Levothyroxine (T4), 116, 118, 119
Levoxyl, 118
Libido. *See* Sex drive
Licorice root, 82, 128
Light therapy, 105, 151
Liver flush cocktail, 56
Liver function, 56–57
Lobster, 100

Magnesium, 94
Many-veggie soup, 66
Medical provider, 38–39
MedQuest, 33
Medroxyprogesterone acetate, 43, 45
Melatonin, 139
Menopause, 12
Mental breaks, 83
Methionine, 56, 128
Methyltestosterone, 43
Migraine headaches, 134–136
Milk thistle, 128
Molecules of Emotion (Candace), 76
Myself system, 138, 151

N-acetyl cysteine, 56
Natural estrogen choices, 52–53
Natural hormones, 3
Natural progesterone, 46
Natural testosterone, 102
Natural vitamin E, 120
Natural vs. synthetic hormones, 42–44
Naturthroid, 119
Negative self-talk, 71
Negative talk, 83
Neuroendocrine, 89
Night sweats, 124–127
Norethindrone acetate, 45

Norris, R. V., 90
Northrup, Christiane, 30
Nutrition. *See* Diet

Oophorectomy, 22
Osteoporosis, 118
Oysters, 100

Pamper yourself, 86
PCOS, 25
Pelvic muscle exercises, 137–138. *See also*
    Kegel exercises
Pencil test, 129
Perimenopause, 1, 12–13, 16–17
Personal time, 82
Pert, Candace, 76
Physical exercise. *See* Exercise
Phytoestrogens, 55, 82
Pineapple, 100
PMS, 9, 87–96
    antidepressants, 96
    assessment, 91–92
    causes, 89–91
    diagnosing, 91–92
    exacerbating/mitigating factors, 91
    products, 151
    progesterone, 95
    supplements, 94–95
    treatment options, 93–96
PMS assessment checklist, 92
Polycystic ovarian syndrome (PCOS), 25
Pre-sleep snacking, 70
Premenstrual syndrome. *See* PMS
Products, 151
Progesterone, 23–24, 52
    administering, 47
    aging, 10
    benefits, 23
    dosage, 47–48
    effect, 49
    estrogen and, 18
    hair loss, 131
    headaches, 135–136
    hot flashes/night sweats, 126
    irregular bleeding, 128
    natural vs. synthetic, 45–47
    need for, 48–49
    normal/optimal range, 37
    PMS, 95

sex drive, 103
  too high/low, 24
  troubleshooting, 49–50
Progesterone capsules, 47, 96
Progesterone creams/gels, 48, 96
Progesterone drops/lozenges, 47–48, 96
Progestin, 45
Prometrium, 46
Protein, 64–65
Protein bars/shakes, 70
Provera, 45

Quick-fix plan
  energy, 121
  stress, 86

Rako, Susan, 102
Raspberries, 100
Raspberry vinaigrette, 67
Recommended reading, 152–154
Recreational activity, 82
Red clover, 126
Relaxation, 80, 114
Replens, 134
Rogaine, 131
Rotterdam Study, 111
Rouzier, Neal, xiii, 32, 33

Salad dressing, 67
Salad tips, 67
Saliva testing, 34, 35
Saw palmetto, 130
Screaming to Be Heard (Vliet), 90
Sears, Barry, 62
Seasonal affective disorder (SAD), 105
Selenium, 120
Self-supportive, 83
Serotonin, 135
Serum testing, 31–33
Sex drive, 97–108
  aphrodisiacs, 100
  barriers to, 106–108
  circulation enhancer, 104
  dream date at home, 108
  exercises, 104, 105
  hormone therapy, 101–102
  lifestyle changes, 104
  light therapy, 105
  products, 151
  sleep, 140
  supplements, 105–106
  testosterone, 102–103
Sex-drive blasters, 106
Sex hormones, 19. *See also* Estrogen;
    Progesterone; Testosterone
Sexual boredom, 108
Sexual fruits, 100
Sex hormone–binding globulin (SHGB), 58
Shames, Richard, 111
Shepherd's purse, 128
Siberian ginseng, 71
Side bends, 105
Simple carbohydrates, 115
Sleep, 114–115, 138–140
Sleep-promoting hormones, 139–140
Smith, Pamela, 64
Snack, 65, 70
Soy supplements, 126
Spironolactone, 93, 130
Strawberries, 100
Stress, 19, 75–86
  adrenal hormones, 77
  busy women, 77–80
  de-stressing, 86, 144
  diet, 85
  exercise, 80, 86
  hair loss, 130
  headaches, 136
  hot flashes/night sweats, 125
  hypothyroidism, 113
  irregular bleeding, 128
  PMS, 91
  quick-fix plan, 86
  solutions, 80–86
  supplements, 82
  symptoms, 80, 81
  working women, 81–83
Stress vitamin, 82
Subclinical hypothyroidism, 110
Sugar, 65
Supplements
  hair loss, 130
  hot flashes/night sweats, 125–127
  hypothyroidism, 120
  irregular bleeding, 128
  PMS, 94–95
  sex drive, 105–106

Supplements *(conintued)*
   sleep, 139
   stress, 82
   weight/fat loss, 71
Synthetic estrogen alternatives, 53–54
Synthetic progesterone, 45
Synthetic vs. natural hormones, 42–44
Synthroid, 118

T3 (Triiodothyronine), 116, 119
T4 (Levothyroxine), 116, 118, 119
T4 L-thyroxine natural, 118
Take Charge of the Change (Smith), 64
Tension headache, 135
Testosterone, 25–26, 38, 99–100
   aging, 10, 101
   benefits, 25, 57
   dosage, 59
   normal/optimal range, 37
   sex drive, 102–103
   things to remember, 58
   too high/low, 25
   vaginal dryness, 133, 134
Testosterone capsules, 59
Testosterone creams/gels, 59
Testosterone drops, 59
Testosterone USP, 102
Thinning hair, 129–131
Thyroid, 110–113
Thyroid 6x, 119
Thyroid 130, 119
Thyroid Glandular, 119
Thyroid hormones, 116
Thyroid Power (Shames), 111
Thyroid R-6, 119
Thyroid-releasing hormone (TRH), 110
Thyroid Solution, The (Arem), 110
Thyroid-stimulating hormone (TSH), 110
Thyroplex, 119
Thyroxine, 118
Topical steroids, 130
Total T3 test, 116
Toxic stress, 78–79. *See also* Stress
TRH, 110
TRH test, 117
Triamcinolone, 130

Tri-estrogen, 52, 53
Triiodothyronine (T3), 116, 119
TSH, 110
TSH test, 116
Tubal ligation, 91
12-week diet overhaul, 143–144
12-week hormonal overhaul, 142–143
Tyrosine, 112, 120

Unithroid, 118
Urine testing, 34

Vacations, 83
Vaginal atrophy, 133
Vaginal dryness, 106, 133–134
Vaginal moisturizers, 134
Valerian root, 139
Vegetables, 66–67
Viagra, 104
Vinaigrettes, 67
Vitamin A, 120
Vitamin C, 120
Vitamin D, 94
Vitamin E, 106, 126, 133
Vitamin E oil, 134
Vitamin/herbal supplement resources,
   149–150
Vliet, Elizabeth Lee, 90

Water, 68, 136, 137
Weight. *See* Body weight
Weight-loss supplements, 151
Westroid, 119
*What Your Doctor May Not Tell You About
   Premenopause* (Lee), 21
Wine, 100
Wisdom of Menopause, The (Northrup), 30
Women's Health Initiative Study, 46
Working women, 81–83. *See also* Busy
   women

Xenohormones, 22

Yogurt cream cheese, 68

Zinc, 55, 82, 120